fMRI in the Pre-Operative Brain Tumor Setting

Editor

ANDREI I. HOLODNY

NEUROIMAGING CLINICS OF NORTH AMERICA

www.neuroimaging.theclinics.com

Consulting Editor
SURESH K. MUKHERJI

February 2021 • Volume 31 • Number 1

ELSEVIER

1600 John F. Kennedy Boulevard • Suite 1800 • Philadelphia, Pennsylvania, 19103-2899

http://www.neuroimaging.theclinics.com

NEUROIMAGING CLINICS OF NORTH AMERICA Volume 31, Number 1
February 2021 ISSN 1052-5149, ISBN 13: 978-0-323-75962-5

Editor: John Vassallo (j.vassallo@elsevier.com)
Developmental Editor: Casey Potter

© 2021 Elsevier Inc. All rights reserved.

This publication and the individual contributions contained in it are protected under copyright by Elsevier, and the following terms and conditions apply to their use:

Photocopying
Single photocopies of single articles may be made for personal use as allowed by national copyright laws. Permission of the Publisher and payment of a fee is required for all other photocopying, including multiple or systematic copying, copying for advertising or promotional purposes, resale, and all forms of document delivery. Special rates are available for educational institutions that wish to make photocopies for non-profit educational classroom use. For information on how to seek permission visit www.elsevier.com/permissions or call: (+44) 1865 843830 (UK)/(+1) 215 239 3804 (USA).

Derivative Works
Subscribers may reproduce tables of contents or prepare lists of articles including abstracts for internal circulation within their institutions. Permission of the Publisher is required for resale or distribution outside the institution. Permission of the Publisher is required for all other derivative works, including compilations and translations (please consult www.elsevier.com/permissions).

Electronic Storage or Usage
Permission of the Publisher is required to store or use electronically any material contained in this periodical, including any article or part of an article (please consult www.elsevier.com/permissions). Except as outlined above, no part of this publication may be reproduced, stored in a retrieval system or transmitted in any form or by any means, electronic, mechanical, photocopying, recording or otherwise, without prior written permission of the Publisher.

Notice
No responsibility is assumed by the Publisher for any injury and/or damage to persons or property as a matter of products liability, negligence or otherwise, or from any use or operation of any methods, products, instructions or ideas contained in the material herein. Because of rapid advances in the medical sciences, in particular, independent verification of diagnoses and drug dosages should be made.

Although all advertising material is expected to conform to ethical (medical) standards, inclusion in this publication does not constitute a guarantee or endorsement of the quality or value of such product or of the claims made of it by its manufacturer.

Neuroimaging Clinics of North America (ISSN 1052-5149) is published quarterly by Elsevier Inc., 360 Park Avenue South, New York, NY 10010-1710. Months of issue are February, May, August, and November. Business and editorial offices: 1600 John F. Kennedy Blvd., Suite 1800, Philadelphia, PA 19103-2899. Business and editorial offices: 6277 Sea Harbor Drive, Orlando, FL 32887-4800. Periodicals postage paid at New York, NY, and additional mailing offices. Subscription prices are USD 397 per year for US individuals, USD 918 per year for US institutions, USD 100 per year for US students and residents, USD 465 per year for Canadian individuals, USD 959 per year for Canadian institutions, USD 541 per year for international individuals, USD 959 per year for international institutions, USD 100 per year for Canadian students and residents and USD 260 per year for foreign students and residents. To receive student/resident rate, orders must be accompanied by name of affiliated institution, date of term, and the *signature* of program/residency coordinator on institution letterhead. Orders will be billed at individual rate until proof of status is received. Foreign air speed delivery is included in all *Clinics* subscription prices. All prices are subject to change without notice. POSTMASTER: Send address changes to *Neuroimaging Clinics of North America*, Elsevier Health Sciences Division, Subscription **Customer Service, 3251 Riverport Lane, Maryland Heights, MO 63043. Telephone: 1-800-654-2452 (U.S. and Canada); 314-447-8871 (outside U.S. and Canada). Fax: 314-447-8029. E-mail: journalscustomerservice-usa@elsevier.com (for print support); journalsonlinesupport-usa@elsevier.com (for online support).**

Reprints. For copies of 100 or more of articles in this publication, please contact the Commercial Reprints Department, Elsevier Inc., 360 Park Avenue South, New York, NY 10010-1710. Tel.: 212-633-3874; Fax: 212-633-3820; E-mail: reprints@elsevier.com.

Neuroimaging Clinics of North America is covered by *Excerpta Medical/EMBASE,* the RSNA Index of Imaging Literature, *MEDLINE/PubMed (Index Medicus),* MEDLINE/MEDLARS, SciSearch, Research Alert, and Neuroscience Citation Index.

PROGRAM OBJECTIVE
The goal of Neuroimaging Clinics of North America is to keep practicing radiologists and radiology residents up to date with current clinical practice in radiology by providing timely articles reviewing the state of the art in patient care.

TARGET AUDIENCE
Practicing radiologists, radiology residents, and other healthcare professionals who utilize neuroimaging findings to provide patient care.

LEARNING OBJECTIVES
Upon completion of this activity, participants will be able to:
1. Review the evolution of functional MRI (fMRI) from research to clinical practice applications.
2. Discuss one of the critical limitations of blood oxygen level dependent (BOLD) fMRI in the setting of focal brain lesions.
3. Recognize the importance of having knowledge of functional neuroanatomy and the role it plays in designing appropriate clinical fMRI paradigms for interpreting study results.

ACCREDITATION
The Elsevier Office of Continuing Medical Education (EOCME) is accredited by the Accreditation Council for Continuing Medical Education (ACCME) to provide continuing medical education for physicians.

The EOCME designates this journal-based CME activity for a maximum of 10 *AMA PRA Category 1 Credit*(s)™. Physicians should claim only the credit commensurate with the extent of their participation in the activity.

All other healthcare professionals requesting continuing education credit for this enduring material will be issued a certificate of participation.

DISCLOSURE OF CONFLICTS OF INTEREST
The EOCME assesses conflict of interest with its instructors, faculty, planners, and other individuals who are in a position to control the content of CME activities. All relevant conflicts of interest that are identified are thoroughly vetted by EOCME for fair balance, scientific objectivity, and patient care recommendations. EOCME is committed to providing its learners with CME activities that promote improvements or quality in healthcare and not a specific proprietary business or a commercial interest.

The planning committee, staff, authors and editors listed below have identified no financial relationships or relationships to products or devices they or their spouse/life partner have with commercial interest related to the content of this CME activity:
Shruti Agarwal, PhD; Behnam Badie, MD; Elham Beheshtian, MD; Nicole Petrovich Brennan, MA; Abbas Chaudhry, PharmD; Ammar A. Chaudhry, MD; Regina Chavous-Gibson, MSN, RN; Melissa M. Chen, MD; Mike Chen, MD, PhD; Gloria C. Chiang, MD; Nicholas S. Cho, BA; Edward J. Ebani, MD; Mohammad M. Fakhri, MD; Madeleine Gene, BS; Sachin K. Gujar, MBBS; Maryam Gul, MD; Andrei I. Holodny, MD, PhD (Hon.), FACR, FASFNR; Rozita Jalilianhasanpour, MD; Rahul Jandial, MD, PhD; Pradeep Kuttysankaran; John J. Lee, MD, PhD; Eric C. Leuthardt, MD; Christie M. Malayil Lincoln, MD; Patrick Luckett, PhD; Alicia Meng, MD; Raquel A. Moreno, MD; Suresh K. Mukherji, MD, MBA, FACR; Sohaib Naim, BSc; Kyung K. Peck, PhD; Jay J. Pillai, MD; Daniel Ryan, MD; Haris I. Sair, MD; Joshua S. Shimony, MD, PhD; Natallia Sopich, MD; Sara B. Strauss, MD; John Vassallo; Kevin Yuqi Wang, MD

UNAPPROVED/OFF-LABEL USE DISCLOSURE
The EOCME requires CME faculty to disclose to the participants:
1. When products or procedures being discussed are off-label, unlabelled, experimental, and/or investigational (not US Food and Drug Administration [FDA] approved); and
2. Any limitations on the information presented, such as data that are preliminary or that represent ongoing research, interim analyses, and/or unsupported opinions. Faculty may discuss information about pharmaceutical agents that is outside of FDA-approved labelling. This information is intended solely for CME and is not intended to promote off-label use of these medications. If you have any questions, contact the medical affairs department of the manufacturer for the most recent prescribing information.

TO ENROLL
To enroll in the *Neuroimaging Clinics of North America* Continuing Medical Education program, call customer service at 1-800-654-2452 or sign up online at http://www.theclinics.com/home/cme. The CME program is available to subscribers for an additional annual fee of USD 265.00.

METHOD OF PARTICIPATION
In order to claim credit, participants must complete the following:
1. Complete enrolment as indicated above.
2. Read the activity.
3. Complete the CME Test and Evaluation. Participants must achieve a score of 70% on the test. All CME Tests and Evaluations must be completed online.

CME INQUIRIES/SPECIAL NEEDS

For all CME inquiries or special needs, please contact elsevierCME@elsevier.com.

NEUROIMAGING CLINICS OF NORTH AMERICA

SERIES OF RELATED INTEREST

Advances in Clinical Radiology
Advancesinclinicalradiology.com
MRI Clinics of North America
Mri.theclinics.com
PET Clinics
pet.theclinics.com
Radiologic Clinics of North America
Radiologic.theclinics.com

THE CLINICS ARE AVAILABLE ONLINE!
Access your subscription at:
www.theclinics.com

NEUROIMAGING CLINICS OF NORTH AMERICA

FORTHCOMING ISSUES

May 2021
Evidence-Based Vascular Neuroimaging
Ajay Malhotra and Dheeraj Gandhi, Editors

August 2021
Imaging of the Thyroid and Parathyroid
Salmaan Ahmed and J. Matthew Debnam, Editors

November 2021
Skull Base Neuroimaging
Stephen Connor, Editor

RECENT ISSUES

November 2020
Machine Learning and Other Artificial Intelligence Applications
Reza Forghani, Editor

August 2020
State of the Art Evaluation of the Head and Neck
Ashok Srinivasan, Editor

May 2020
Magnetoencephalography
Roland R. Lee and Mingxiong Huang, Editors

SERIES OF RELATED INTEREST

Advances in Clinical Radiology
Neuroimaging Clinics
MRI Clinics of North America
PET Clinics
Radiologic Clinics of North America
Radiologic Clinics

THE CLINICS ARE NOW AVAILABLE ONLINE!
Access your subscription at:
www.theclinics.com

Contributors

CONSULTING EDITOR

SURESH K. MUKHERJI, MD, MBA, FACR
Clinical Professor, Marian University, Director
of Head and Neck Radiology, ProScan
Imaging, Regional Medical Director, Envision
Physician Services, Carmel, Indiana, USA

EDITOR

**ANDREI I. HOLODNY, MD, PhD (Hon.),
FACR, FASFNR**
Founding President of the ASFNR, Chief of the
Neuroradiology Service, Director of the
Functional MRI Laboratory, Department of
Radiology, Memorial Sloan Kettering Cancer
Center, Professor of Radiology, Weill Medical
College of Cornell University, Professor of
Neuroscience, Weill Cornell Graduate School
of Medical Sciences, New York, New York,
USA

AUTHORS

SHRUTI AGARWAL, PhD
Research Associate, Division of
Neuroradiology, The Russell H. Morgan
Department of Radiology and Radiological
Science, Johns Hopkins School of Medicine,
Baltimore, Maryland, USA

BEHNAM BADIE, MD
Division Chief and Professor, Department of
Neurosurgery, City of Hope National Cancer
Center, Los Angeles, California, USA

ELHAM BEHESHTIAN, MD
Research Fellow, Division of Neuroradiology,
The Russell H. Morgan Department of
Radiology and Radiological Science, Johns
Hopkins School of Medicine, Baltimore,
Maryland, USA

NICOLE PETROVICH BRENNAN, MA
The New School for Social Research, New
York, New York, USA

ABBAS CHAUDHRY, PharmD
Post-doctoral Fellow, Department of
Diagnostic Radiology, City of Hope National
Cancer Center, Los Angeles, California, USA

AMMAR A. CHAUDHRY, MD
Director, Precision Imaging Lab, Associate
Director of Imaging Informatics Research,
Assistant Professor, Department of Diagnostic
Radiology, City of Hope National Cancer
Center, Los Angeles, California, USA

MELISSA M. CHEN, MD
Assistant Professor, Department of Diagnostic
Radiology, Division of Diagnostic Imaging, The
University of Texas MD Anderson Cancer
Center, Houston, Texas, USA

MIKE CHEN, MD, PhD
Associate Professor, Department of
Neurosurgery, City of Hope National Cancer
Center, Los Angeles, California, USA

GLORIA C. CHIANG, MD
Associate Professor, Department of Radiology, Division of Neuroradiology, Weill Cornell Medical Center, New York, New York, USA

NICHOLAS S. CHO, BA
Medical Scientist Training Program, David Geffen School of Medicine at UCLA, Los Angeles, California, USA

EDWARD J. EBANI, MD
Diagnostic Radiology Resident, Department of Radiology, Weill Cornell Medical Center, New York, New York, USA

MOHAMMAD M. FAKHRI, MD
Mallinckrodt Institute of Radiology, Washington University, St Louis, Missouri, USA

MADELEINE GENE, BS
Department of Radiology, Memorial Sloan Kettering Cancer Center, New York, New York, USA

SACHIN K. GUJAR, MBBS
Assistant Professor, Division of Neuroradiology, The Russell H. Morgan Department of Radiology and Radiological Science, Johns Hopkins School of Medicine, Baltimore, Maryland, USA

MARYAM GUL, MD
Assistant Professor, Department of Diagnostic Radiology, City of Hope National Cancer Center, Los Angeles, California, USA

ANDREI I. HOLODNY, MD, PhD (Hon.), FACR, FASFNR
Founding President of the ASFNR, Chief of the Neuroradiology Service, Director of the Functional MRI Laboratory, Department of Radiology, Memorial Sloan Kettering Cancer Center, Professor of Radiology, Weill Medical College of Cornell University, Professor of Neuroscience, Weill Cornell Graduate School of Medical Sciences, New York, New York, USA

ROZITA JALILIANHASANPOUR, MD
Research Fellow, Division of Neuroradiology, The Russell H. Morgan Department of Radiology and Radiological Science, Johns Hopkins School of Medicine, Baltimore, Maryland, USA

RAHUL JANDIAL, MD, PhD
Associate Professor, Department of Neurosurgery, City of Hope National Cancer Center, Los Angeles, California, USA

JOHN J. LEE, MD, PhD
Mallinckrodt Institute of Radiology, Washington University, St Louis, Missouri, USA

ERIC C. LEUTHARDT, MD
Department of Neurological Surgery, Washington University School of Medicine, St Louis, Missouri, USA

CHRISTIE M. MALAYIL LINCOLN, MD
Assistant Professor, Department of Radiology, Baylor College of Medicine, Houston, Texas, USA

PATRICK LUCKETT, PhD
Department of Neurology, Washington University School of Medicine, St Louis, Missouri, USA

ALICIA MENG, MD
Neuroradiology Fellow, Department of Radiology, Weill Cornell Medical Center, New York, New York, USA

RAQUEL A. MORENO, MD
Department of Radiology, Memorial Sloan Kettering Cancer Center, New York, New York, USA; Instituto do Câncer do Estado de São Paulo (ICESP), São Paulo-SP, Brazil

SOHAIB NAIM, BSc
Research Associate, Department of Diagnostic Radiology, City of Hope National Cancer Center, Los Angeles, California, USA

KYUNG K. PECK, PhD
Departments of Medical Physics, and Radiology, Memorial Sloan Kettering Cancer Center, New York, New York, USA

JAY J. PILLAI, MD
Director of Functional MRI, Associate Professor of Radiology and Neurosurgery, Division of Neuroradiology, The Russell H. Morgan Department of Radiology and Radiological Science, Department of Neurosurgery, Johns Hopkins School of Medicine, Baltimore, Maryland, USA

DANIEL RYAN, MD
Instructor, Division of Neuroradiology, The
Russell H. Morgan Department of Radiology
and Radiological Science, Johns Hopkins
School of Medicine, Baltimore, Maryland,
USA

HARIS I. SAIR, MD
Associate Professor, Director of
Neuroradiology, Division of Neuroradiology,
The Russell H. Morgan Department of
Radiology and Radiological Science, Johns
Hopkins School of Medicine, The Malone
Center for Engineering in Healthcare, The
Whiting School of Engineering, Johns Hopkins
University, Baltimore, Maryland, USA

JOSHUA S. SHIMONY, MD, PhD
Mallinckrodt Institute of Radiology,
Washington University, St Louis, Missouri, USA

NATALLIA SOPICH, MD
Department of Radiology, Memorial Sloan
Kettering Cancer Center, New York, New York,
USA

SARA B. STRAUSS, MD
Neuroradiology Fellow, Department of
Radiology, Weill Cornell Medical Center, New
York, New York, USA

KEVIN YUQI WANG, MD
Resident, Department of Radiology, Baylor
College of Medicine, Houston, Texas, USA

Contents

> During the past decade, functional MR imaging has rapidly moved from the research environment into clinical practice. Preoperative functional MR imaging is now standard clinical practice not only in major academic institutions, but also in community neurosurgical and neuroradiologic practices. The clinical use of functional MR imaging will only increase in the years to come. Application of functional MR imaging (including resting-state functional MR imaging) to the context of neuropsychiatric diseases is likely to continue to advance.

> Functional magnetic resonance imaging (fMRI) is useful for localizing eloquent cortex in the brain prior to neurosurgery. Language and motor paradigms offer a wide range of tasks to test brain regions within the language and motor networks. With the help of fMRI, hemispheric language dominance can be determined. It also is possible to localize specific motor and sensory areas within the motor and sensory gyri. These findings are critical for presurgical planning. The most important factor in presurgical fMRI is patient performance. Patient interview and instruction time are crucial to ensure that patients understand and comply with the fMRI paradigm.

> There are many technical and nontechnical steps involved in a successful clinical functional MRI (fMRI) scan. The output from scanning and analysis can only be as good as the input, so task instruction and rehearsal are the most important steps during an clinical fMRI procedure. Properly pre-processed data significantly affects statistical analysis, which has a great impact on image interpretation. Even though there is general agreement on how to process clinical fMRI data, such as algorithms for head motion detection and correction, the theory and practicalities associated with data processing remain complex and constantly evolving.

> Knowledge of functional neuroanatomy is essential to design the most appropriate clinical functional MR imaging (fMR imaging) paradigms and to properly interpret

unique insight into preoperative planning for central nervous system (CNS) neoplasms by identifying areas of the brain effected or spared by the neoplasm. BOLD (blood-oxygen-level–dependent) fMR imaging can be reliably used to map eloquent cortex presurgically and is sufficiently accurate for neurosurgical planning. In patients with brain tumors undergoing neurosurgical intervention, fMR imaging can decrease postoperative morbidity. This article discusses the applications, significance, and interpretation of BOLD fMR imaging, and its applications in presurgical planning for CNS neoplasms.

Radiographic monitoring of posttreatment glioblastoma is important for clinical trials and determining next steps in management. Evaluation for tumor progression is confounded by the presence of treatment-related radiographic changes, making a definitive determination less straight-forward. The purpose of this article was to describe imaging tools available for assessing treatment response in glioblastoma, as well as to highlight the definitions, pathophysiology, and imaging features typical of true progression, pseudoprogression, pseudoresponse, and radiation necrosis.

In 2016, the World Health Organization (WHO) central nervous system (CNS) classification scheme incorporated molecular parameters in addition to traditional microscopic features for the first time. Molecular markers add a level of objectivity that was previously missing for tumor categories heavily dependent on microscopic observation for pathologic diagnosis. This article provides a brief discussion of the major 2016 updates to the WHO CNS classification scheme and reviews typical MR imaging findings of adult primary CNS neoplasms, including diffuse infiltrating gliomas, ependymal tumors, neuronal/glioneuronal tumors, pineal gland tumors, meningiomas, nerve sheath tumors, solitary fibrous tumors, and lymphoma.

Foreword

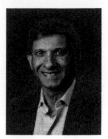

Suresh K. Mukherji, MD, MBA, FACR
Consulting Editor

This issue of *Neuroimaging Clinics* focuses on the fascinating field of functional MR imaging (fMR imaging). I remember my complete amazement when I first saw the brain "think" on MR images. One of the fun things I routinely do is give a talk to a high-school anatomy class on neuroradiology, and it is really cool to see their excitement when I show the fMR images.

The promise of fMR imaging has been around for decades, and I am eagerly awaiting the day when the Nobel Prize is awarded to those that helped develop this powerful technique. The transition of fMR imaging into clinical practice has progressed at a deliberate pace. The majority of clinical and research studies are performed at academic centers and other large health care organizations. Part of the challenge has been to define the clinical applications that can be translated into our daily practice. This has been facilitated by the development of a separate CPT code for fMR imaging.

This was the rationale and goal for this issue of *Neuroimaging Clinics*, and I would like to thank

Dr Andrei Holodny for guest editing this important issue. I would also like to thank all of the authors for their wonderful contributions. This edition reviews various fMR imaging techniques and has specific articles dedicated to various clinical applications in central nervous system oncology and presurgical planning. I am sure this multidisciplinary issue will provide a better understanding of fMR imaging and its clinical applications.

Suresh K. Mukherji, MD, MBA, FACR
Clinical Professor, Marian University
Director of Head and Neck Radiology
ProScan Imaging
Regional Medical Director
Envision Physician Services
Carmel, Indiana, USA

E-mail address:
sureshmukherji@hotmail.com

Neuroimag Clin N Am 31 (2021) xv
https://doi.org/10.1016/j.nic.2020.09.013
1052-5149/21/© 2020 Published by Elsevier Inc.

Preface
Functional MR Imaging: Ready for Clinical Prime Time

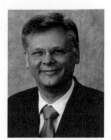

Andrei I. Holodny, MD, PhD (Hon.), FACR, FASFNR
Editor

Functional MR imaging (fMR imaging) has clearly revolutionized the imaging and understanding of the human brain. Within the past few years, this powerful technology has advanced into the clinical arena, not only in major academic centers but also into small-group private practices. At the present time, fMR imaging (or an analogous method, such as magnetoencephalography or transcranial magnetic stimulation) should be part of the preoperative workup in patients with brain tumors or seizure disorders. The transition of fMR imaging into clinical practice has been facilitated by the development of a separate CPT code for fMR imaging, the founding of the American Society of Functional Neuroradiology (ASFNR) as well as numerous courses on this topic.

However, even though fMR imaging is an exceptionally powerful technology that can significantly influence how a neurosurgeon approaches a brain tumor, there are a number of vagaries of fMR imaging that need to be acknowledged in order to optimally perform and interpret this examination. Probably the most important aspect of fMR imaging is the need for the person performing the fMR imaging examination to interact with the patient both before and during the scan to optimize study. Properly preparing the patient to perform the required paradigm in the scanner or adjusting said paradigm based on the patient's underlying neurologic condition is often the difference between success and failure. This feature of fMR imaging can also serve as an opportunity for the radiologist to interact with the patient and demonstrate his/her clinical relevance.

Looking into the future, as our understanding of the function of the brain in health and pathology increases, and as MR technology and computer methods improve, it is my firm belief that the clinical applicability of fMR imaging will only grow. This progress will probably occur in the areas of resting state fMR imaging and in neurocognitive and neuropsychiatric disorders, including children and the elderly. Such progress will serve to make neuroradiology even more scientifically exciting and clinically irreplaceable.

I would like to thank the authors of the articles in this issue, who are world-class leaders the field of fMR imaging.

My fervent hope, dear reader, is that the volume that you hold in your hands will assist you in your exciting journey of applying this wonderful, powerful, and ever-evolving technology to the benefit of your patients.

Andrei I. Holodny, MD, PhD (Hon.), FACR, FASFNR
Department of Radiology
Memorial Sloan-Kettering Cancer Center
1275 York Avenue
New York, NY 10065, USA

E-mail address:
holodnya@mskcc.org

Website:
http://www.mskcc.org/cancer-care/doctor/andrei-holodny

Neuroimag Clin N Am 31 (2021) xvii
https://doi.org/10.1016/j.nic.2020.09.012
1052-5149/21/© 2020 Published by Elsevier Inc.

Introduction to Functional MR Imaging

Natallia Sopich, MD, Andrei I. Holodny, MD*

KEYWORDS

• Functional MRI (fMRI) • fMRI data analysis • Paradigm selection

KEY POINTS

- Functional MR imaging is an outstanding clinical test that has already moved into routine clinical practice.
- To optimize functional MR imaging results, the person administering the functional MR imaging must ensure that the patient performs the paradigm correctly.
- It is important to understand the pitfalls of functional MR imaging, including susceptibility artifacts, the significance of the P value, and the effect of neovasculature.
- To correctly interpret functional MR imaging studies, one must understand the physics of MR imaging, appreciate each patient's neuroanatomy, and look for evidence of cortical reorganization.

INTRODUCTION

In the past decade, functional MR imaging (fMR imaging) has rapidly moved from the research environment into clinical practice. Preoperative fMR imaging is now standard clinical practice not only in major academic institutions but also in community neurosurgical and neuroradiologic practices. Functional MR imaging has been endorsed by the American Academy of Neurology.[1] So far, the most common clinical application of fMR imaging has been in preoperative planning for patients with brain tumors or seizures.

In brain tumor surgery, the neurosurgeon aims to maximize resection of the brain tumor while avoiding resection of eloquent cortices, which could lead to loss of essential functions such as language and movement. In this setting, the neurologic functions of most concern to the neurosurgeon are the motor and speech functions. fMR imaging is a useful tool to identify the eloquent cortices preoperatively (and, with the use of neurosurgical navigational systems, intraoperatively). Three-dimensional visualization of the anatomic relationship of the tumor to adjacent eloquent cortices makes preoperative planning and the resection of the brain tumor more manageable for the neurosurgical team.[2–4]

If you were a neurosurgeon, which image presented in **Fig. 1** would you prefer to use in preoperative planning? Would you prefer the left image (radiologic right), in which a probable low-grade tumor seems to be situated somewhere at the frontoparietal junction (does it involve the motor cortex?), or the right image (radiologic left), in which the relationship of the tumor to the cortex is clearly visible? Let us consider how useful images such as the right image are obtained.

WHAT IS FUNCTIONAL MR IMAGING?

Functional MR imaging is a brain mapping technique that allows clinicians to identify eloquent

---

Funding information: National Institutes of Health (NIH): NIH-NIBIB R01 EB022720 (Makse and Holodny, PIs), NIH-NCI R21 CA220144 (Holodny and Peck, PIs), NIH-NCI U54 CA137788 (Ahles, PI), NIH-NCI P30 CA008748 (Thompson, PI).
Department of Radiology, Memorial Sloan Kettering Cancer Center, 1275 York Avenue, New York, NY 10065, USA
* Corresponding author.
E-mail address: holodnya@mskcc.org

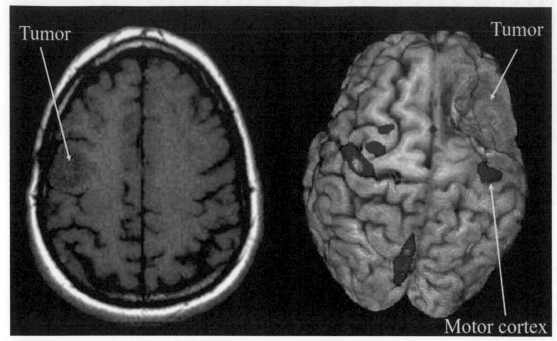

Tumor   Tumor

Motor cortex

Fig. 1. Anatomic MR imaging (*left*) versus fMR imaging (*right*). If you were a referring physician, which image would you prefer to use to help you make crucial presurgical decisions?

cortex on anatomic MR images. Eloquent cortex is defined as an area of gray matter essential for the performance of functions such as sensation, movement, speech, vision, and higher cortical functions, including memory. Functional MR imaging provides a closer look at the brain, but determines precisely (well, nearly precisely) which part of the brain handles each function.

Functional MR imaging visualizes and measures the quick and small metabolic changes that take place in an active part of the brain. Signal intensity changes occur in each voxel of the brain over time as patients perform specific tasks (fMR imaging paradigms).

HOW ARE FUNCTIONAL MR IMAGING DATA ACQUIRED?

> *If you can't explain it to a six-year-old, you don't understand it well enough.*
> —Albert Einstein

Functional MR imaging was first described by Seiji Ogawa in 1990. He called his technique blood oxygen level dependent (BOLD) fMR imaging because it uses oxyhemoglobin and deoxyhemoglobin in the blood vessels as an endogenous contrast agent to generate functional activation maps.[5]

BOLD fMR imaging is based on the following principle: an increase in neuronal activity causes an increase in local oxygen extraction from the blood because of an increase in the cerebral metabolic rate of oxygen. This increase leads to an increase in paramagnetic deoxyhemoglobin, which lowers the signal intensity. However, after several seconds, neuronal activity also causes an increase in cerebral blood flow and cerebral blood volume, which leads to an increase in the flow of oxygenated blood and an increase in oxyhemoglobin. For yet unknown reasons, the amount of oxygenated blood that arrives to support the active neurons far exceeds the metabolic need. This overcompensation of oxyhemoglobin leads to a decrease in the ratio of deoxyhemoglobin to oxyhemoglobin, which is measurable and is the basis for BOLD fMR imaging signal (**Figs. 2** and **3**).

Following the advice of professor Einstein, we can also offer the flowing explanation in case, dear reader, you might have the need to explain what you do to nonscientists, perhaps curious children or grandchildren (with perfuse apologies to the physicists among the readership). We all know that different parts of the brain control different functions. When a part of brain starts "working"—for example, the part of the brain that controls the movement of the fingers when I move my right hand—more blood flows to that area of the brain. Everyone knows that when

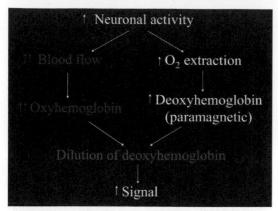

Fig. 2. Schemata of the generation of BOLD signal demonstrating the relationship between increased neuronal activity and increased BOLD signal through manipulation of oxyhemoglobin and deoxyhemoglobin.

they run, more blood flows to their legs. Blood contains red blood cells, red blood cells contain hemoglobin, hemoglobin contains iron, and iron is a little magnet—everyone knows this. Hence, when a part of the brain starts working harder, more "small magnets" flow to this area, which can be seen by the "magnetic" resonance scanner (MR imaging). And we have just explained the very complicated process of fMR imaging in a very understandable way!

The basic scheme for acquiring fMR imaging data and incorporating it into brain surgical practice is depicted in **Box 1**.

HOW DOES FUNCTIONAL MR IMAGING ACQUISITION DIFFER FROM ANATOMIC MR IMAGING ACQUISITION?

During the acquisition of routine brain scans, we assume that the signal intensity in each voxel does not change over time. In contrast, the basis of fMR imaging is that the signal intensity changes over the time of the acquisition as the patient performs a certain task (or paradigm).

Anatomic MR imaging sequences typically take 3 to 4 minutes to acquire, whereas fMR imaging scans the whole brain very quickly (typically 1–4 seconds) multiple times during the acquisition to capture the signal intensity changes over short periods of time. The long acquisition time of anatomic MR imaging enables the acquisition of high-resolution images with a matrix of 256×256 or higher; fMR imaging images are typically acquired using a 64×64 matrix.

The simplest fMR imaging paradigm is known as a "boxcar paradigm," during which the patient performs a task and then rests. This "on" (task period) and "off" (rest period) sequence is repeated a number of times (**Fig. 4**).

HOW ARE FUNCTIONAL MR IMAGING DATA ANALYZED?

After data acquisition, the next step is to produce an fMR imaging map. To do so, one must analyze which voxels are "active" based on the paradigm administered during fMR imaging acquisition.

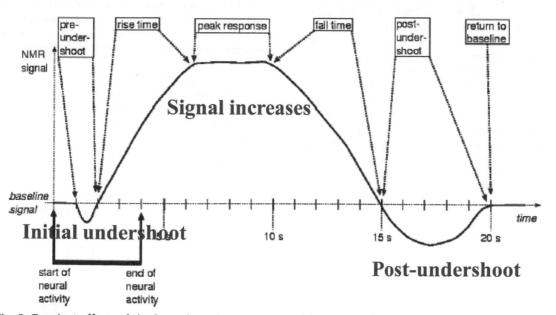

Fig. 3. Transient effects of the hemodynamic response. Local increase in deoxygenated blood (paramagnetic) leads to brief metabolic negative BOLD effect (initial undershoot). Large influx of oxygenated blood (diamagnetic) produces the fMR imaging T2* signal (signal increases).

Box 1

Basic scheme for acquiring fMR imaging data and incorporating this data into presurgical planning in the brain tumor setting

1. Functional MR imaging data
2. High resolution (T1+Gd, fluid attenuation inversion recovery, etc)
3. Analyze fMR imaging data offline
4. Co-register fMR imaging data with T1 data
5. Load onto neurosurgical computer

Voxels that are active during the stimulus period and inactive during the rest period are likely being used to perform the task.

From the fMR imaging data, a signal intensity curve is generated over time for each voxel in the brain. This signal intensity–time curve is then compared with the stimulus to determine if there is a correlation between the two. There are many different statistical ways to determine the correlation, which range from simple to very complex. A commonly used method is to determine if there is a correlation between the signal change in a specific voxel and the timing of the paradigm. (For more on methods of analysis, please see Peck and colleagues' article, "Methods of Analysis: Functional MR imaging for Pre-surgical Planning," in this issue.)

If a signal correlates significantly with the paradigm for a specific voxel, that voxel is considered active. **Fig. 4** presents a patient who was asked as part of his fMR imaging paradigm to alternate moving his tongue and resting. The patient's tongue movement is depicted by the red line. When the patient moves his tongue, the red line elevates to 1; when he rests, the red line returns to zero. The blue line represents the signal change over time (**Fig. 5**). In the top graph, the BOLD signal changes in concert with the patient's tongue movement; when the patient moves his tongue, the signal increases. When he rests, the signal reverts to baseline. This voxel corresponds with the known location of the motor homunculus of the tongue. This voxel is considered active and is

depicted in yellow. The lower graph depicts a voxel that has nothing to do with tongue movement. Visual inspection demonstrates that there is no correlation between the BOLD signal (in blue) and the paradigm (in red). Therefore, this voxel is not considered active. Simply put, an fMR imaging map is a correlational map of signal intensity changes in the fMR imaging paradigm.

There are several types of fMR imaging paradigm:

1. *Motor:* Foot, hand, face, and tongue movement
2. *Sensory:* Sensory stimulation (can also be used as a motor paradigm if the patient has motor weakness)
3. *Language:* Category, letter, verb generation, sentence completion, and number counting
4. Visual
5. Auditory
6. Memory
7. Higher cortical function

These paradigm types are described in greater detail in later articles.

CHALLENGES OF FUNCTIONAL MR IMAGING

To successfully acquire and accurately read fMR imaging results, one must understand its challenges: susceptibility artifacts, P value, and the effect of neovasculature.

Susceptibility artifacts (signal dropout) can be caused by dental work, blood products, hemosiderin from a previous surgery, or infarct. Dropout artifacts from the air–tissue interface at the base of the brain are also common in patients with brain tumors. As a result, T2* source images should be routinely inspected to determine if susceptibility artifacts are present.[6]

Most commercial and noncommercial statistical analysis tools allow the user to vary parameters such as the correlation coefficient or P value. The challenge is that there is no universally accepted P value. In everyday clinical practice, one usually adjusts the P value until the image "looks right," or until the area of interest is clearly visible and activity in other areas is minimized. For purists, this may seem to be scientifically unsatisfactory;

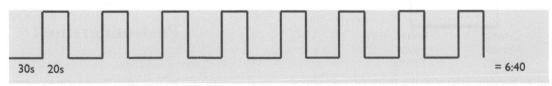

30s   20s   = 6:40

Fig. 4. Example of paradigm design: repeated 20 sec blocks of activity separated by 30-second blocks of rest (6–8 cycles total).

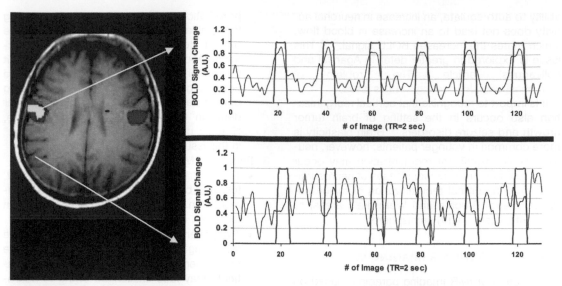

Fig. 5. Motor tongue paradigm and signal intensity in significant versus not significant voxels.

however, this method generally answers the clinical question at hand, for example, identifying Broca's area in relation to a tumor as part of presurgical planning.

Abnormal tumor neovasculature can lead to a decrease in BOLD fMR imaging signal. The BOLD signal depends on a predictable vascular response, but as tumor neovasculature loses the

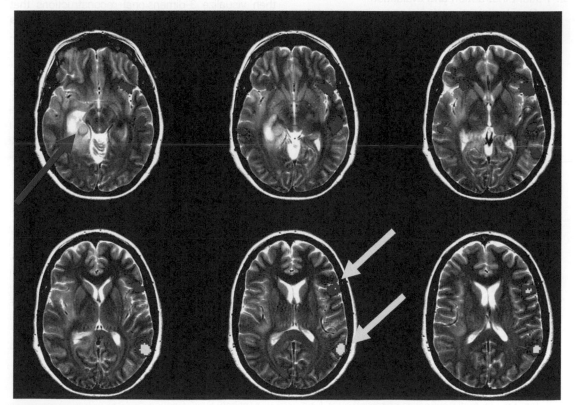

Fig. 6. The lesion to be resected is seen in the right temporal lobe (*red arrow*). Functional MR imaging demonstrated that the patient was left language dominant. The *yellow arrows* show Broca's and Wernicke's areas. Based on this information, the neurosurgeon was able to complete the procedure with the patient under total anesthesia and was able to resect the lesion without an iatrogenic language deficit.

ability to autoregulate, an increase in neuronal activity does not lead to an increase in blood flow, which mutes the increased BOLD signal.[7–11] This issue is explored in greater detail in Agarwal and colleagues' article, "The Problem of Neurovascular Uncoupling," in this issue.

It is import to recognize that cortical reorganization also occurs in the setting of brain tumor growth and seizure disorders.[12] Brain plasticity is more common in younger patients; however, neurosurgically significant reorganization may occur into adulthood. This includes cases of neurosurgically proven cortical reorganization of major language areas (Broca's and Wernicke's areas) to the contralateral (right) hemisphere.[13–16]

THE FUNCTIONAL MR IMAGING WORKFLOW

1. Selection of fMR imaging paradigm based on area of interest
   - Surgeon refers patient and gives brief history of neurologic deficit. The neuroradiologist reviews images to determine lesion location and chooses fMR imaging paradigm targeted to lesion location.
2. Patient instruction and evaluation
   - Good patient performance is essential to achieve optimal fMR imaging results. The most important aspects of patient preparation are interviewing and assessing the clinical status of the patient, giving the patient detailed pre-fMR imaging instructions, modifying the paradigm practice to fit the patient's abilities and limitations, and answering any clinical questions. Optimizing patient performance is discussed in greater detail in Brennan and colleagues' article, "Patient preparation and paradigm design," in this issue.
3. Functional MR imaging and data acquisition
   - The fMR imaging should be acquired first, followed by the anatomic MR imaging (high-resolution T1+Gd, fluid attenuation inversion recovery, etc).
   - The patient should be monitored during the fMR imaging examination to ensure that he or she performs the paradigm correctly. Patients may face challenges owing to neurologic impairments or difficulty understanding or following instructions. Patients may become tired or may accidently move.

The co-registered images can be downloaded to the neurosurgical computer. The neurosurgeon can then visualize 3-dimensional reconstructions that define the relationship between the lesion and the eloquent cortices to guide the brain tumor resection.

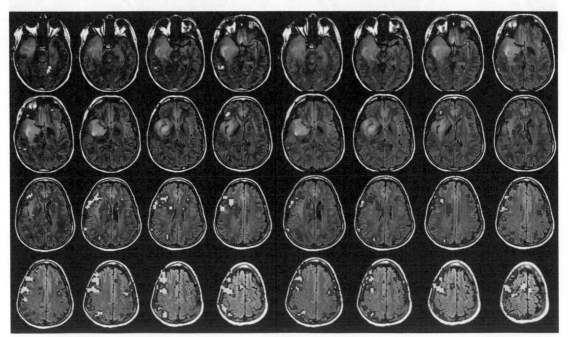

Fig. 7. The lesion to be resected is seen in the right temporal lobe. However, in this case, in contradistinction from Fig. 6, fMR imaging demonstrated that the patient was right language dominant (ipsilateral to the lesion). This information necessitated the neurosurgeon to perform the operation "awake" and to use DCS to identify language areas intraoperatively.

CLINICAL USEFULNESS OF FUNCTIONAL MR IMAGING

The primary clinical application of fMR imaging has been preoperative brain tumor surgery planning. In this context, it is essential to maximize the resection of the lesion while avoiding the adjacent eloquent cortex to minimize postoperative deficits. Preoperative identification of eloquent cortices could help neurosurgeons to decide whether to perform a resection, biopsy, or not to operate at all; to choose the best surgical approach; to plan the extent of the resection; and to decide how best to perform intraoperative direct cortical stimulation (DCS).

Often, the most important question for the neurosurgeon is whether or not the lesion to be resected is ipsilateral or contralateral to the dominant language areas. Intraoperative DCS remains the gold standard in localizing the dominant language areas; however, this procedure is time consuming and may be difficult to perform. During DCS, the patient awakes from general anesthesia and is asked to perform task-based paradigms (eg, language tests) while the surgeon or neurophysiologist stimulates the brain with electrodes to elicit the appropriate response. For example, the location in which DCS elicits speech arrest defines the location of the essential language cortex. To further complicate matters, this test is performed while the patient is extubated; hence, certain parameters such as blood oxygenation are difficult to control. Taking these limitations into consideration, fMR imaging data demonstrating that the lesion to be resected are contralateral to the major language areas and that the patient can forego DCS is quite useful to the neurosurgeon. In the case presented in **Fig. 6**, the patient is clearly left language dominant, and the lesion to be resected is on the right side of the brain. The neurosurgeon was able to complete the procedure with the patient under total anesthesia and was able to resect the lesion without an iatrogenic language deficit. In contrast, the

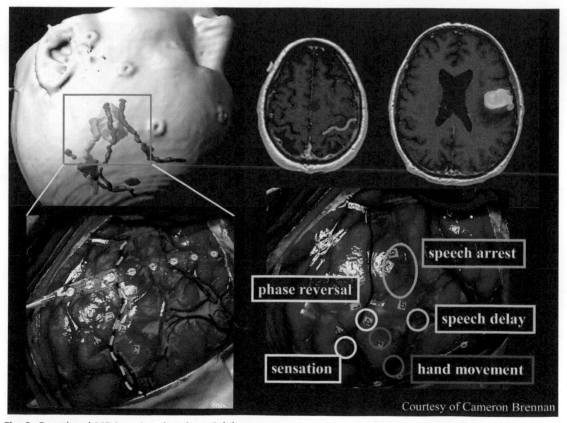

Courtesy of Cameron Brennan

Fig. 8. Functional MR imaging data (*top right*) was reconstructed in 3 dimensions and overlaid on the image of the patient's head using the angulation that the neurosurgeon would see during his/her approach to the tumor. Green indicates the central sulcus, the location of which was derived from fMR imaging results identifying the motor strip (*red*). *Yellow* indicates the tumor. *Purple lines* indicate overlying veins. The location of these structures was confirmed intraoperatively (*bottom right*).

patient presented in **Fig. 7** also had a lesion on the right side of the brain, but fMR imaging demonstrated that the patient was right language dominant. Hence, before resection, DCS was necessary to identify the language areas intraoperatively.

Once language laterality is established, the neurosurgeon must determine the anatomic relationship of the lesion to adjacent eloquent areas. Unexpected challenges may arise owing to natural atypical organization or tumor-induced reorganization of eloquent areas. Tumor masses may displace or even split functional areas, and eloquent areas may move ipsilaterally or contralaterally owing to cortical plasticity. These topics are explored in greater detail in subsequent articles.

Functional MR imaging results can be manipulated to optimize visualization of essential cortical structures, including 3-dimensional displays to guide resection (**Fig. 8**). In addition to preoperative planning, fMR imaging can be incorporated into the neurosurgical navigational system to guide the operation (**Fig. 9**).

To summarize, preoperative fMR imaging has several distinct advantages:

1. Allows better preoperative planning
2. Noninvasive (vs DCS)
3. Decreases intraoperative "surprises"
4. Decreases time of operation and time under anesthesia
5. Sometimes intraoperative mapping does not work—problems with sedation or the deep sulci cannot be adequately mapped
6. Can be used multiple times without risk (vs PET)

OTHER CLINICAL APPLICATIONS AND NOVEL DIRECTIONS OF FUNCTIONAL MR IMAGING

The clinical usefulness of fMR imaging is not limited to brain tumors: fMR imaging has been applied in several other contexts, including diagnosis of neurodegenerative diseases such as Alzheimer's disease (AD), Parkinson disease, dementia with Lewy bodies (DLB), and frontotemporal dementia; psychiatric conditions such as schizophrenia, bipolar disorder, depression,

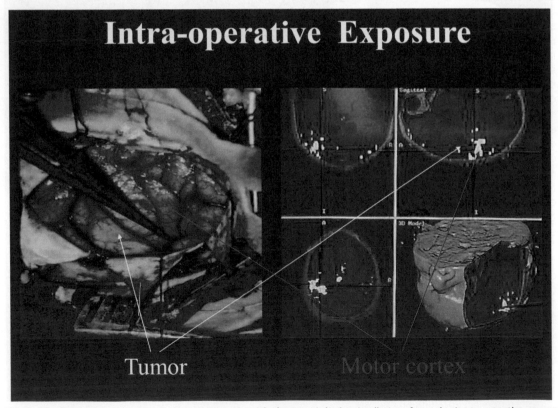

Fig. 9. The intraoperative view (*left*) corresponds with the top right (sagittal) view from the intraoperative screen capture of the neuro-navigational system (*right*). It is impossible to discern the location of the motor strip by viewing the exposed brain. The *red crosshairs* depict the location of the tip of the pointer. The low signal intensity structure anterior to the tip of the pointer marks the location of the tumor. *White voxels* depict the location of the motor strip (just posterior to the tip of the pointer).

suicidal ideation, memory decline, autism, attention deficit and hyperactivity disorder, and dyslexia; as well as multiple sclerosis, stroke, mild traumatic brain injury, epilepsy, and many more.[17]

AD is a major health concern in the United States and will become more severe as the population ages in the coming years. Many pharmaceutical treatments target patients with mild cognitive impairment rather than advanced disease. Functional MR imaging can demonstrate decreased activity in areas of the brain adversely affected by AD and increased activity in compensatory areas. A key to AD treatment is to identify AD before the patient develops debilitating symptoms. Several recent studies have used fMR imaging to demonstrate changes in patients with mild cognitive impairment from AD or before the development of AD symptoms. For instance, a recent fMR imaging study by Julie K. Wisch and colleagues[18] revealed changes in intranetwork connections in patients with AD nearly 4 years before clinical disease presentation, thus demonstrating that fMR imaging findings may be a useful biomarker of brain health.

In Parkinson disease, the second-most widespread neurodegenerative disorder, functional rearrangements of the basal ganglia–thalamus–motor cortex connectivity have been found to show higher neurofunctional coupling between the prefrontal cortex and striatum and lower coupling between the pallidum, subthalamic nucleus, and paracentral lobule.[19] One study demonstrated that an increase in motor impairment is associated with a decrease in the motor activation of the posterior putamen.[20] Thus, fMR imaging could be an important tool for the early identification and prediction of Parkinson disease and for evaluating neurofunctional changes caused by therapeutic agents and neurorehabilitation strategies.[21]

Functional MR imaging also raises important diagnostic biomarkers for another common cause of dementia—DLB. Alterations in several functional networks have been found in patients with DLB when compared with healthy controls and patients with AD.[22] In patients with DLB, higher activation has been identified in the basal ganglia network and reduced activation has been identified in the default mode and salience and executive networks.

A recent study of patients with schizophrenia demonstrated a correlation between aberrations in functional connectivity and reduced gray matter volumes, as well as increased functional connectivity between sensorimotor–precuneus–parietal areas and frontal–temporal–insular cortices.[23]

Likewise, fMR imaging techniques play an important role in our comprehension of underlying biological aspects of depression and have identified new subtypes by distinguishing patterns of dysfunctional connectivity that could guide therapy approaches and help develop new treatment strategies,[24,25] including prediction of antidepressant response owing to pretreatment differences in intrinsic functional brain networks.[26]

Understanding functional brain connectivity is important not only to understand health and disease, but also to understand how specific skills affect cognitive processes that can be used to guide treatment. For example, a study evaluated the effect of chess playing on whole brain functioning and found increased brain network fluidity in chess experts compared with beginners; thus, the researchers hypothesized that "gaming" could improve cognitive processes and could be used as a medication by clinicians.[27]

Another interesting study revealed an inverse correlation between length of education and symptom severity in patients with frontotemporal dementia.[28] This investigation concluded that patients with the same clinical severity but with more years of education have worse functional brain alterations, suggesting that higher cognitive capability causes higher cognitive reduction.

DISCLOSURE

N. Sopich has nothing to disclose. A.I. Holodny is the Owner/President of fMR imaging Consultants, LLC, a purely educational entity.

REFERENCES

1. Szaflarski JP, Gloss D, Binder JR, et al. Practice guideline summary: use of fMRI in the presurgical evaluation of patients with epilepsy: report of the Guideline Development, Dissemination, and Implementation Subcommittee of the American Academy of Neurology. Neurology 2017;88:395–402.
2. Gupta A, Shah A, Young RJ, et al. Imaging of brain tumors: functional magnetic resonance imaging and diffusion tensor imaging. Neuroimaging Clin N Am 2010;20(3):379–400.
3. Gabriel M, Brennan NP, Peck KK, et al. Blood oxygen level dependent functional magnetic resonance imaging for presurgical planning. Neuroimaging Clin N Am 2014;24(4):557–71.
4. Brennan NPPK, Holodny A. Language mapping using fMRI and direct cortical stimulation for brain tumor surgery: the good, the bad, and the questionable. Top Magn Reson Imaging 2016;25:1–10.

5. Ogawa S, Lee TM, Kay AR, et al. Brain magnetic-resonance-imaging with contrast dependent on blood oxygenation. Proc Natl Acad Sci U S A 1990;87(24):9868–72.

6. Peck KK, Bradbury M, Petrovich N, et al. Presurgical evaluation of language using functional magnetic resonance imaging in brain tumor patients with previous surgery. Neurosurgery 2009;64(4):644–52.

7. Chen CM, Hou BL, Holodny AI. Effect of age and tumor grade on BOLD functional MR imaging in preoperative assessment of patients with glioma. Radiology 2008;248(3):971–8.

8. Holodny AI, Schulder M, Liu WC, et al. Decreased BOLD functional MR activation of the motor and sensory cortices adjacent to a glioblastoma multiforme: implications for image-guided neurosurgery. AJNR Am J Neuroradiol 1999;20(4):609–12.

9. Holodny AI, Schulder M, Liu WC, et al. The effect of brain tumors on BOLD functional MR imaging activation in the adjacent motor cortex: implications for image-guided neurosurgery. AJNR Am J Neuroradiol 2000;21(8):1415–22.

10. Fraga de Abreu VHPK, Petrovich-Brennan NM, Woo KM, et al. Brain tumors: the influence of tumor type and routine MR imaging characteristics at BOLD functional MR imaging in the primary motor gyrus. Radiology 2016;281:876–83.

11. Sun H, Vachha B, Laino ME, et al. decreased hand motor resting-state functional connectivity in patients with glioma: analysis of factors including neurovascular uncoupling. Radiology 2020;294(3):610–21.

12. Fisicaro RA, Jost E, Shaw K, et al. Cortical plasticity in the setting of brain tumors. Top Magn Reson Imaging 2016;25(1):25–30.

13. Holodny AI, Schulder M, Ybasco A, et al. Translocation of Broca's area to the contralateral hemisphere as the result of the growth of a left inferior frontal glioma. J Comput Assist Tomogr 2002;26(6):941–3.

14. Petrovich NM, Holodny AI, Brennan CW, et al. Isolated translocation of Wernicke's area to the right hemisphere in a 62-year-man with a temporoparietal glioma. AJNR Am J Neuroradiol 2004; 25(1):130–3.

15. Mallela AN, Peck KK, Petrovich-Brennan NM, et al. Altered resting-state functional connectivity in the hand motor network in glioma patients. Brain Connect 2016;6(8):587–95.

16. Li Q, Dong JW, Del Ferraro G, et al. Functional translocation of Broca's area in a low-grade left frontal glioma: graph theory reveals the novel, adaptive network connectivity. Front Neurol 2019;10: 1664–2295.

17. Valsasina P, Hidalgo de la Cruz M, Filippi M, et al. Characterizing rapid fluctuations of resting state functional connectivity in demyelinating, neurodegenerative, and psychiatric conditions: from static to time-varying analysis. Front Neurosci 2019;13: 1662–4548.

18. Wisch JK, Roe CM, Babulal GM, et al. Resting state functional connectivity signature differentiates cognitively normal from individuals who convert to symptomatic Alzheimer's disease. J Alzheimers Dis 2020;74(4):1085–95.

19. Akram H, Wu C, Hyam J, et al. l-Dopa responsiveness is associated with distinctive connectivity patterns in advanced Parkinson's disease. Movement Disord 2017;32(6):874–83.

20. Herz DM, Eickhoff SB, Lokkegaard A, et al. Functional neuroimaging of motor control in Parkinson's disease: a meta-analysis. Hum Brain Mapp 2014; 35(7):3227–37.

21. Filippi M, Sarasso E, Agosta F. Resting-state functional MRI in parkinsonian syndromes. Mov Disord Clin Pract 2019;6(2):104–17.

22. Lowther ER, O'Brien JT, Firbank MJ, et al. Lewy body compared with Alzheimer dementia is associated with decreased functional connectivity in resting state networks. Psychiatry Res Neuroimaging 2014;223(3):192–201.

23. Abrol A, Rashid B, Rachakonda S, et al. Schizophrenia shows disrupted links between brain volume and dynamic functional connectivity. Front Neurosci 2017;11:1662–4548.

24. Lynch CJ, Gunning FM, Liston C. Causes and consequences of diagnostic heterogeneity in depression: paths to discovering novel biological depression subtypes. Biol Psychiatry 2020;88(1): 83–94.

25. Drysdale AT, Grosenick L, Downar J, et al. Resting-state connectivity biomarkers define neurophysiological subtypes of depression. Nat Med 2017;23: 28–38.

26. Dunlop K, Talishinsky A, Liston C. Intrinsic brain network biomarkers of antidepressant response: a review. Curr Psychiatry Rep 2019;21(9):87.

27. Premi E, Gazzina S, Diano M, et al. Enhanced dynamic functional connectivity (whole-brain chronnectome) in chess experts. Sci Rep 2020;10(1): 7051.

28. Premi E, Cristillo V, Gazzina S, et al. Expanding the role of education in frontotemporal dementia: a functional dynamic connectivity (the chronnectome) study. Neurobiol Aging 2020;93:35–43.

Patient Preparation and Paradigm Design in fMRI

Madeleine Gene, BS[a], Nicole Petrovich Brennan, MA[b], Andrei I. Holodny, MD[a],*

KEYWORDS

- fMRI • Brain tumors • Gliomas • Language paradigms • Motor paradigms • Patient preparation

KEY POINTS

- Clinical functional magnetic resonance imaging (fMRI) is useful for localizing eloquent cortex in the brain prior to neurosurgery.
- With the help of fMRI, hemispheric language dominance can be determined, and Broca area, Wernicke area, and secondary language areas can be localized.
- The specific motor and sensory areas within the motor and sensory gyri also can be localized.
- The most important factor in presurgical fMRI is patient performance. It is crucial to be generous with patient interview and instruction time to ensure that patients understand and comply with the fMRI paradigm.

INTRODUCTION

Preoperative functional magnetic resonance imaging (fMRI) in patients with brain tumors or seizure disorder has moved into the clinical arena.[1,2] Clinical fMRI is very different from basic fMRI, however, and requires a specialized and dedicated approach.[3] Unlike healthy volunteers for basic science research, patients in need of fMRI often present with significant impairments that complicate the examination. Developing patient-specific fMRI paradigms and extensively preparing patients for the scan are necessary to mitigate the effects of patient impairment. Thus, the most important aspect of fMRI administration occurs before a patient even gets in the scanner.

SCAN PREPARATION

Proper preparation is crucial to successful administration of clinical fMRI. When an ordering physician requests an fMRI examination, 4 pieces of information must be collected. These data should inform the approach taken in each case.

Age

There are documented differences in fMRI performance[4] and blood oxygen–level dependent (BOLD) response[5–10] between older and younger patients. Older patients may produce more head motion; patient age and motion have been positively correlated.[4] Care must be taken to emphasize the importance of keeping the head still. Older patients show fewer activated voxels and greater noise in activated voxels, resulting in reduced signal-to-noise ratios.[5] Several studies have shown that the BOLD response is lower in amplitude in older adults than in younger adults,[7–10] which may reflect differences in neurovascular coupling.[9] Working with older patients may require additional instruction or in-scanner guidance to mitigate contamination of the BOLD response with noise or motion artifact. Using aural and visual stimulation simultaneously during fMRI tasks may help these patients successfully complete the examination.

On the opposite end of the age spectrum, pediatric fMRI also requires additional preparation. The most common reasons for failure in pediatric

[a] Department of Radiology, Memorial Sloan Kettering Cancer Center, 1275 York Avenue, New York, NY 10065, USA; [b] The New School for Social Research, 80 Fifth Avenue, New York, NY 10011, USA
* Corresponding author.
E-mail address: holodnya@mskcc.org

Neuroimag Clin N Am 31 (2021) 11–21
https://doi.org/10.1016/j.nic.2020.09.007
1052-5149/21/© 2020 Elsevier Inc. All rights reserved.

scans include excessive head motion, insufficient instruction, and fear of the noise or confinement of the scanner. Younger children generally are less successful with fMRI.[11] Children younger than age 8 years have shown significantly lower success rates than children over age 8 years.[12] Even so, in-scanner head motion (relative mean displacement [mm]) may be 4 times higher in a patient aged 8 years compared with a patient aged 20 years. The effect of age on head motion seems to decrease with age.[13] It is important to consider the particular challenges of scanning pediatric patients. Familiarizing children with the magnetic resonance imaging machine, providing ample instruction, and practicing before the scan may improve the quality of the results.

Handedness

The handedness of patients is important to consider when interpreting language fMRI cases. Many studies have shown that more than 90% of right-handed individuals (often as many as 95%) show left hemispheric (typical) dominance for language.[14–16] Among left-handed individuals, however, as few as 74% show typical left dominance. The incidence of bilateral language activation also is higher among left-handed than among right-handed people.[17] There may be a linear relationship between the degree of laterality and degree of handedness, with higher incidence of right hemispheric (atypical) dominance among the strongly left-handed than among the ambidextrous and strongly right-handed.[15,17–19]

Because a relationship has been observed between handedness and language dominance, it is important to collect this information from the patient. Knowing a patient's handedness informs interpretation of the fMRI results. For instance, if patients are left-handed, it is more likely that they show atypical language activation. The most common tool used to assess handedness is the Edinburgh Handedness Inventory.[20] This measurement includes information about hand preference for everyday activities, including writing, drawing, and using scissors. Some older naturally left-handed patients may have been trained to predominately use the right hand.[21] These forced right-handed individuals may show different functional neuroanatomy than naturally right-handed individuals.[22]

Deficits

Because impairment can severely limit a patient's ability to perform fMRI tasks, it is crucial to identify patient deficits prior to scan administration. Brain tumor patients may suffer from neurologic symptoms, including dysphasia, paresis, forgetfulness, confusion, and anxiety. Patients also may suffer from claustrophobia and may need premedication. Modifying existing paradigms is essential to accommodate many of these limitations.[23,24] A patient with hand or foot paresis likely will struggle to perform assigned motor tasks. In this case, the paradigm can be modified to apply external sensory stimulation to the affected area. This can be used to produce motor activation despite a patient's motor impairment.[25,26] A patient with dysphasia or aphasia likely will have difficulty with standard language paradigms. Slowing the timing of the paradigm or reducing the frequency of stimulation can help improve patient performance. It also may be helpful to select the simplest task from the battery of language paradigms.[27] Gathering information about functional impairment from either the patient or the ordering physician allows the fMRI to be tailored to each patient. Modifying the paradigm to suit each patient's individual abilities gives the patient a greater chance of success.

Tumor Type and Location

When working with brain tumor patients, it is crucial to consider a patient's cancer diagnosis and lesion location. High-grade gliomas, such as glioblastoma multiforme, may increase the risk of false-negative results. This is thought to occur through neurovascular uncoupling, in which the tumor disrupts normal neovasculature, such that an increase in neuronal activity does not lead to an increase in blood flow.[10,28–31] Because fMRI relies on normal BOLD response, disruption of the normal neovascular response can result in reduced fMRI activation.[23,24,29] The radiologist interpreting the fMRI data in such cases must consider the risk of false negatives. The person administering the fMRI examination also must be aware of this risk to monitor the fMRI results effectively in real time.

Gliomas can alter the expected fMRI response due to cortical plasticity.[32–34] Because low-grade gliomas grow more slowly than high-grade gliomas, these tumors may be more prone to functional reorganization.[35–37] This slow rate of tumor expansion, as opposed to acute injury, may allow the brain to slowly reorganize and develop compensatory mechanisms.[37] Intrahemispheric and interhemispheric reorganization both have been observed,[37,38] with activation seen in local preserved cortices and analogous contralateral structures, respectively. The possibility of functional reorganization may explain why most patients with low-grade gliomas show normal or nearly normal neurologic examinations.[36] In such cases, when the left Broca area is invaded, for example, atypical right Broca activation may reflect compensatory activation.[39] It, therefore, is important to consider how a patient's diagnosis may affect the fMRI results, particularly when the results are unexpected.

Finally, the tumor location should inform paradigm selection. When a tumor is close to eloquent cortex, functional paradigms designed to activate that cortex should be performed (eg, language paradigms for tumors close to Broca area). Choosing appropriate paradigms based on different clinical scenarios is discussed later.

PATIENT EVALUATION
Patient Interview

Successful clinical fMRI requires detailed prescan patient preparation. This component of the examination requires interviewing, evaluating, and instructing the patient.[23,24,26,27] The interview often begins by assessing the patient's clinical status, including asking about any deficits. The patient's handedness also is determined. It is critical to evaluate the function that will be tested during the fMRI examination to ensure that the patient will be able to perform the task.[24] As discussed previously, it is essential to modify any existing functional paradigms to accommodate patient limitations.

For a hand motor paradigm, for example, hand weakness must be tested for prior to the scan. For a language paradigm, the patient's productive or receptive speech must be tested. The authors use the Boston Naming Test, a subtest of the Boston Diagnostic Aphasia Examination, to evaluate productive speech. The Boston Naming Test contains 60 standardized line drawings that the patient is asked to name, organized in order of word frequency.[40] Auditory responsive naming questions describing concepts (eg, "name a big animal with a trunk") may be used to test the patient's receptive speech ability.[41] Informal assessment through conversation also can provide evidence of possible deficit.

After the patient is evaluated, the procedure is explained to the patient in detail. This explanation should familiarize the patient with the task and the paradigm timing, including how the in-scanner instructions will be administered (ie, visually or aurally). For example, the patient should be told to expected to be still for 30 seconds and then tap fingers for 20 seconds, repeating this sequence 8 times. It is advisable to do a brief trial run of the selected task to maximize compliance in the scanner.[24,26] The patient's success or lack thereof in the prescan rehearsal also can serve as a predictor of patient performance. If there are special circumstances, such as a visual impairment, hearing difficulty, or language barriers, these should be addressed during the prescan interview.[23,27] If a patient is receiving contrast, nursing staff should insert the intravenous line at this time.

The patient should arrive at least 1 hour before the scheduled scan to complete these tasks.[23] This preparatory time spent with the patient can make the difference between a strong fMRI map and an uninterpretable one. Adequate patient preparation and evaluation are essential.

LANGUAGE

fMRI paradigms should be selected based on a patient's clinical scenario. These should include a thorough review of prior imaging and an evaluation of patient symptoms. Because the goal of presurgical fMRI is to identify eloquent cortex for the benefit of the neurosurgeon, the paradigms selected must seek to activate brain regions in close proximity to the lesion.[23] This section focuses on paradigms designed to activate the language areas of the brain based on functional neuroanatomy. There are several situations in which it is appropriate to perform language fMRI paradigms.

It is important to identify hemispheric language dominance in cases where language areas are impacted. As discussed previously, most right-handed individuals display typical left hemisphere language dominance. In right-handed patients, language paradigms, therefore, are appropriate for most left hemisphere lesions; they also are appropriate for right hemisphere lesions when a patient displays aphasia. Because it is highly unlikely that a right-handed patient shows right hemisphere language dominance, it usually is unnecessary to perform language paradigms in these cases unless clinically indicated (aphasia). For left-handed and ambidextrous people, language paradigms are appropriate for lesions in both hemispheres.

Language Functional Neuroanatomy

The language network is composed of several essential primary language areas and additional secondary language areas. Although there may be variability among individuals in precise anatomic localization,[42,43] the frontal lobe generally controls productive speech and the temporoparietal lobes generally control receptive speech.[26]

Primary Language Areas

Classically, the main productive speech area in the frontal lobe is known as Broca area. This area, located within the inferior frontal gyrus, and more specifically within the pars opercularis and pars triangularis (Brodmann areas 44 and 45), is essential for expressive language.[44] Damage to this area can produce Broca aphasia, a nonfluent aphasia characterized by telegraphic, dysarthric, or agrammatic speech, or even mutism in severe cases.[24,26,45] Patients may have difficulty with object naming, word fluency, and other productive components of speech[46]; however, comprehension commonly remains intact with insult to Broca area.[26] Direct cortical stimulation (DCS) of this region during an awake craniotomy can produce total speech arrest.[3,47] Therefore, neurosurgeons commonly order fMRI examinations when there is tumor in the vicinity of Broca area.

Wernicke area, the main receptive speech area, is located in the posterior superior temporal gyrus posterior to the Heschl (auditory) gyrus.[3,24] This region classically has been considered the main area for language comprehension in the brain. As opposed to frontal lobe dysfunction, patients with temporal lobe dysfunction tend to present with varied language deficits.[3] Injury to the Wernicke area can result in phonemic paraphasia (eg, substituting "pike" for "pipe"), semantic paraphasia (eg, substituting "train" for "car"), fluent aphasia (eg, word salad), circumlocution, or word-finding difficulty.[24,26,48] Patients also may exhibit symptoms of receptive aphasia, including an inability to understand commands or answer questions. The varied nature of Wernicke aphasia aligns with DCS findings showing high variability of the localization of language function within the temporoparietal region.[3] In 1 study in which DCS was performed on the temporal lobe, only 30.6% of patients showed a temporal lobe language site.[43] Wernicke area may also play a role in perceptual, integrative, and verbal memory functions.[3]

Broca and Wernicke areas are part of the classic model of language (the Wernicke–Geschwind model). Recent work suggests that the simple distinction between areas of speech production and speech comprehension may not reflect the true nature of language processing in the brain. Many researchers favor a more complex view.[49–53] Yet identifying Broca and Wernicke areas still is useful in presurgical clinical fMRI. Modern models of language postulate that several language areas play a supportive role in the language network. These brain regions are called secondary language areas.

Secondary Language Areas

One well-known secondary language area is the middle frontal gyrus (MFG).[3,48,54,55] This region, also known as the dorsolateral prefrontal cortex, is located superior to Broca area. Language fMRI tasks can produce strong activation of the MFG that is comparable to Broca area in degree of lateralization.[54] For example, strong left-sided Broca area activation may be accompanied by strong left-sided MFG activation, which supports left hemispheric dominance. The MFG is important for verbal working memory as well as cognition and information integration.[48] DCS of the MFG infrequently produces language disturbance (approximately 10%)[43,48]; however, dysarthria and anomia both have been observed with insult to the region.[3] When resections have resulted in postoperative language deficits, these deficits generally have been temporary.[48,49]

The supplementary motor area (SMA), despite its name, also plays a supportive role in language function. The SMA is located in the medial superior frontal gyrus, with the foot motor homunculus located just posteriorly.[3] The SMA consists of 2 functional subdivisions, known as the pre-SMA (anterior-most portion of the SMA) and the SMA proper (posterior to the pre-SMA).[3,48] The pre-SMA and SMA proper are thought to support language and motor planning, respectively. There also is evidence of a central SMA, with joint motor and language function.[56,57] Resection of the SMA is known to produce SMA syndrome, a transient postoperative disorder characterized by a paucity of speech or akinetic mutism.[48] Strangely, SMA syndrome often resolves on its own within weeks to months.[51,58] A patient is at 100% risk of developing SMA syndrome when a tumor is within 5 mm of the SMA.[59] Resection of tumors in the SMA typically is considered safe due to the transient nature of the resulting postoperative deficits.[51]

Another area of interest is the insula; however, this region's role in language is not well understood. This is in part because it is a relatively deep structure, located deep to the frontal operculum.[3,48] A meta-analysis of fMRI studies has implicated the insula in several different components of language, showing similar insular activation for both receptive and expressive speech.[60] This region likely plays a role in end-stage speech production (articulation)[61,62] and ventilation during speech.[63] It also may play a part in naming, word-finding, and articulation.[64] Damage to the insula may produce variable language deficits or none at all. Speech apraxia has been correlated with insult to the region.[62] Damage to the insula alone is rare, which has made it difficult to draw conclusions about the region's role in language.[63] Although this region is not a target for presurgical fMRI, insular activation frequently is seen during language tasks.[3]

The final language areas to consider are the supramarginal and angular gyri, which together comprise the inferior parietal lobule. The supramarginal gyrus is located anterior to the upturned aspect of the sylvian fissure, whereas the angular gyrus surrounds the posterior aspect of the sylvian fissure.[3] Although the function of the angular gyrus is not well defined,[48] a meta-analysis has shown that the angular gyrus frequently activates during semantic processing.[65] The region may support reading, in particular.[66,67] On the other hand, the supramarginal gyrus may contribute to phonological processing[68] and verbal working memory.[48] There are limited surgical data for these 2 regions; however, the angular gyrus is related to alexia and agraphia,[69] and the supramarginal gyrus is related to anomia and slurred/slowed speech.[70] fMRI typically is not used to sensitively predict deficits based on the location of the inferior parietal lobule; rather, identifying reading-associated cortices often occurs via DCS during neurosurgery.[3]

This discussion of primary and secondary language areas should serve as an introduction to the functional neuroanatomy of the language network. These areas can be expected to be seen to activate during language fMRI tasks. The greater understanding of the brain regions of interest, the more successful the presurgical fMRI.

LANGUAGE PARADIGMS
Paradigm Design

The fMRI paradigms selected should target the brain region of interest. The most common type of paradigm design is a block design, which consists of alternating active and resting blocks. For example, for a hand motor task, the patient alternates between 20 seconds of hand movement and 30 seconds of hand relaxation for several repeating cycles. Averaging the signal from at least 5 to 6 of these cycles increases statistical power and produces a stronger fMRI signal. On the other hand, event-related paradigms also consist of active and resting blocks but instead are designed to capture the neural response after a single stimulus event. These paradigms are composed of much shorter stimulus periods, usually less than 4 seconds long, with many more repetitions. Because block paradigms produce a strong average signal with greater statistical

power, this design is preferred in patients for clinical fMRI.[23,24,26]

Frontal Paradigms

Language paradigms should target productive (frontal) and receptive (temporoparietal) speech areas.[24,27] It is important to perform multiple language paradigms per language case to confirm the accuracy of the results (preferably 2 to 3).[55] A lesion in the frontal lobe requires frontal speech mapping. For these cases, tasks involving word generation, such as semantic and phonemic fluency, frequently are performed. Semantic fluency tasks present the patient with a letter and ask the patient to generate words that begin with the given letter. Phonemic fluency tasks present the patient with a category (eg, animals, colors, or vegetables) and ask the patient to generate words belonging to that category.[23,26] Another paradigm used to activate productive frontal areas is the verb generation task. This paradigm presents patients with a noun and asks patients to generate verbs associated with that noun. For example, for the noun "baby," patients would generate words, such as "eats," "sleeps," "cries," and "crawls."[24] The verb generation task produces results with greater specificity and less variability in hemispheric dominance than other tasks, perhaps because it requires more complex language processing.[3] These productive speech tasks generally elicit activation of the receptive speech areas as well.[55]

Temporoparietal Paradigms

Lesions in the temporoparietal lobes typically target the Wernicke area. This region often is more difficult to measure than the frontal region, even when using tasks specifically designed for receptive speech.[3,23] Language mapping for these lesions generally requires comprehension tasks, such as reading, listening, and sentence completion.[24,26] During the sentence completion task, the patient reads a sentence in which the final word has been replaced with a blank line. The patient must generate a word that logically completes the sentence.[23] This task can be administered visually or aurally. When administered visually, it is possible to implement a button response with 4 possible answer choices. For example, "Bill gives haircuts and shampoos. He is a _____ (1) butcher (2) barber (3) batch (4) beer."[3] Another possible receptive task is auditory responsive naming. Patients listen to simple questions, such as "What do you shave with?" and

"What color is grass?" and generate the answers to these questions.[3]

Notes on Paradigms

Overlearned sequences, such as number counting, should be avoided in language mapping. Compared with object naming, number counting is a less sensitive task for both language localization and lateralization. Number counting has been shown to yield fewer areas of speech interruption during DCS than object naming, which may be due to the task's simple, overlearned nature.[71] Using one of the tasks, discussed previously, produces more reliable results. In certain cases, however, in which the patient has severe language deficits, number counting may be the only paradigm that the patient is able to perform. In the authors' clinical practice, clinically meaningful fMRI language studies have been able to be acquired in such circumstances.

The fMRI patient typically is asked to generate responses silently (covert) rather than vocalize them (overt). Silent word generation during language tasks helps to minimize motion artifact due to vocalization; however, covert responses make it impossible to monitor patient performance aurally.[27] Nevertheless, covert paradigms are suggested alongside real-time fMRI analysis to monitor patient performance.[24]

Most fMRI paradigms elicit activation from both frontal and temporoparietal language areas. Despite attempts to isolate productive and receptive speech with specific tasks, many language paradigms activate Broca and Wernicke areas equally.[23,24,27] It is possible to adapt most, if not all, language tasks to either aural or visual paradigm delivery. For some patients, one method works better than the other (eg, in cases of visual or hearing impairment). Aural delivery may allow for more dynamic administration of the examination, which is useful when adapting to patients' limitations during the scan. On the other hand, visual delivery may produce more consistent results.[72]

Lateralization

An essential goal of presurgical language mapping is to determine hemispheric language dominance. Intracarotid amobarbital testing (Wada testing) is considered the gold standard for determining language lateralization.[72] During Wada testing, one of the brain's hemispheres is anesthetized in order to test language function in the other.[73] fMRI is a less invasive alternative to Wada testing because it does not involve sedation. Several studies have determined concordance between Wada and fMRI testing to be in the range of 86% to 91%.[74–76] Discordance between the 2 methods may be caused by variability in fMRI acquisition, paradigms, and analysis, which can result in language maps of varying quality. Regardless, the high concordance and lower risk of fMRI have led many centers to embrace fMRI for presurgical language mapping.[73]

MOTOR

As with language fMRI paradigms, motor fMRI paradigms must be selected based on a patient's clinical scenario. This requires review of the patient's symptoms and prior imaging to determine if the lesion impinges on eloquent motor cortex.[24] Even if the motor cortex is not impacted directly, if a patient has motor or sensory deficits, it may be helpful to perform motor paradigms for the affected area (ie, hands, face, and so forth.). For some language cases, it also may be necessary to use motor paradigms to identify the tongue motor area.

Motor Functional Neuroanatomy

The primary motor cortex (M1) is essential for movement, and the primary somatosensory cortex (S1) is essential for sensation. Both motor and sensory systems are organized topographically; the motor and sensory functions of different body parts are located in specific locations along the precentral and postcentral gyri. These maps of motor and sensory function along the cortex are known as the motor homunculus and sensory homunculus, respectively. In the motor homunculus, the foot and leg motor areas are located along the interhemispheric fissure. The hand motor area is lateral to the foot motor area, and the tongue and face motor areas are lateral to the hand motor area.[24–26]

The SMA is composed of the pre-SMA and the SMA proper, the latter of which is involved in motor planning and also is known to support word articulation.[24] Because motor paradigms are necessary when a lesion impinges on the SMA, many patients undergo motor mapping to localize this region. This is important because the anatomic boundaries of the SMA are not well defined,[26] which puts patients at risk for SMA syndrome.[77]

The organization of the motor and sensory regions must be understood to properly plan for each fMRI, because tasks must be chosen based on the motor homunculus. More specifically, determining the location of the lesion within the motor strip determines which motor tasks should be performed. For example, a patient with a lesion in or near the tongue area of the primary motor cortex needs to perform a tongue motor task. Patients with lesions close to the midline should perform foot motor tasks, whereas patients with lesions close to the reverse omega portion of the central sulcus (the hand motor area) should perform hand motor tasks.[23]

Ultimately, the purpose of fMRI motor mapping is to identify the motor areas that have a close anatomic relationship with the lesion.[24,26] Such motor mapping also is helpful when anatomy is ambiguous or effaced due to the presence of a lesion; the neuroradiologist may be able to identify the precentral and postcentral gyri in these cases with the help of fMRI.

Foot Motor

When the foot motor area is impacted, identifying the foot motor activation is critically important. Losing foot mobility can render a patient wheelchair-bound or bedbound. The foot motor task requires patients to wiggle the toes by performing toe flexion and extension. This task is somewhat difficult to perform without introducing movement, because patients often move the entire body in the z (inferior to superior) direction when wiggling the toes.[26] Care must be taken to instruct the patient to isolate movement to the feet and toes. An alternative is to ask the patient to tap the feet against one another in the x and y directions (perpendicular to the long axis of the body). This also decreases motion in the z direction.

Hand Motor

The hand motor (finger-tapping) task requires patients to tap their thumbs to each finger sequentially while minimizing other body movements.[24] If patients suffer from distal hand weakness, they can perform a modified version of the task in which patients simply open and close the hands (fist clenching).[24,26] If a patient is too weak to complete the modified motor task, passive hand simulation should be performed. When a patient has weakness in 1 hand, the activation map may be asymmetric. It often is useful to perform the motor task first with both hands and then with the affected hand alone in order to focus on the affected hemisphere.

Tongue and Face Motor

To elicit tongue motor activation, patients are asked to keep the mouth closed and to sweep the tongue against the back of the teeth, taking care to avoid head motion.[24] Only a slight amount of movement is necessary to activate the tongue motor area because the tongue, mouth, and lips take up a relatively large portion of the motor homunculus.[26] If lip or face motor activation is of interest, patients are asked to purse the lips and push them back into a smile, repeatedly. Locating the tongue and lip motor areas often takes place with language mapping.

Passive Stimulation

As discussed previously, when a patient is too weak to perform the hand or foot motor task, passive sensory stimulation must be applied in the form of brushing, squeezing, or touching the hand or foot.[25] It has been shown that passive stimulation is a valid alternative or complement to active motor paradigms.[78] Passive stimulation also is useful when a patient is unable to follow the paradigm instructions or complete the motor task without excessive head motion. Alternatively, if the postcentral gyrus is impacted or if a patient suffers from numbness, performing sensory paradigms may be useful. Although sensory paradigms activate the postcentral (sensory) gyrus, they often activate both motor and sensory areas.[24,26] Because such reciprocity exists between motor and sensory areas,[25] the results of these tasks must be interpreted with caution.

SCAN SET-UP

After assessing the patient's clinical situation and completing the prescan interview, the final step before administering the fMRI is setting the patient up in the scanner.

Which type of paradigm delivery system to use during the scan must be decided. For visual delivery, a back projection and mirror may be used. A sophisticated set of noise-canceling headphones and liquid crystal display goggles for visual delivery also can be purchased.[23] For aural delivery, instructions can be delivered to patients through headphones or in-room speakers. As a last resort, if other methods fail, the magnetic resonance (MR) room can be entered and the patient's leg or arm simply tapped to indicate "start" and "stop." It is essential to test the system prior to beginning the scan. The patient must be able to hear what is being said through the headphones and see what is being presented visually on the screen or goggles.

It is important to remind the patient that the scan is extremely sensitive to motion and that head motion must be minimized. Ensuring that the patient is in a comfortable position in the scanner increases compliance and reduce motion.[23,24] The patient can be made more comfortable by putting a pillow under the knees and providing a blanket. Patients also should use the restroom before the scan begins so that they are able to complete the entire study without pause. This is true especially for children. Patients must stay in the same position for the entire study, even when the scanner is not acquiring images, so that the fMRI images can be coregistered onto the high-resolution postcontrast T1-weighted images.[23] To make this possible, patients must minimize all motion.

Once a scan begins, it is useful to speak to the patient through the headphones between sequences.[26] A small amount of encouragement can go a long way. Because the fMRI paradigm is not intuitive to most patients, reiterating instructions immediately before each task can increase compliance. In addition, reassurance that they are performing the task correctly may improve patients' performance.[26] Between each sequence, the task also can be clarified or adjusted as needed.

Monitoring patient performance is an important part of administering the fMRI examination. For example, if a patient is asked to perform finger-tapping, the patient must be watched to ensure that the patient actually moves the fingers. If the patient fails to perform the task, the results are meaningless.[23] Most MR machines allow the operator to monitor fMRI activity in real time. This is a useful tool for monitoring patient performance, especially for covert language tasks, which are restricted to the patient's mind. If the language regions are visible on this raw map, there can be fair confidence in the quality of the fMRI results.[24]

SUMMARY

Clinical fMRI is a useful tool for localizing eloquent cortex in the brain prior to neurosurgery. Language and motor paradigms offer a wide range of tasks to test specific brain regions in the language and motor networks. With the help of fMRI, hemispheric language dominance can be determined and Broca area, Wernicke area, and secondary language areas can be localized. It also is possible to localize specific motor and sensory areas in the motor and sensory gyri. These findings are critical for presurgical planning. The most important factor in presurgical fMRI is patient performance. Sophisticated fMRI devices and software offer little benefit if time is not taken to prepare for the scan, examine the patient, explain the procedure, make any necessary adjustments, and monitor the patient throughout the examination. It is crucial to be generous with the interview and instruction time to ensure that the patient understands and complies with the fMRI paradigms. With proper patient instruction and paradigm selection, the battle for quality fMRI results already is half-won.

CLINICS CARE POINTS

- Pre-operative brain tumor patients often neurologically compromised and may have difficulty understanding or performing the fMRI paradigm.
- A neurological examination and patient preparing the before the fMRI scan is essential.
- The most important determinate of a successful fMRI examination is patient cooperation.
- Monitoring the patient during the fMRI examination to ensure compliance with the paradigm will increase the number of fMRI studies of diagnostic quality.

ACKNOWLEDGMENTS

Funding support provided by the National Institutes of Health (NIH): NIH-NIBIB R01 EB022720 (Makse and Holodny, PI's); NIH-NCI R21 CA220144 (Holodny and Peck, PI's); NIH-NCI U54 CA137788 (Ahles, PI); and NIH-NCI P30 CA008748 (Thompson, PI).

DISCLOSURE

N.P. Brennan and M. Gene have nothing to disclose. A. Holodny is the Owner/President of fMRI Consultants, LLC, a purely educational entity.

REFERENCES

1. Gupta A, Shah A, Young RJ, et al. Imaging of brain tumors: functional magnetic resonance imaging and diffusion tensor imaging. Neuroimaging Clin N Am 2010;20(3):379–400.
2. Gabriel M, Brennan NP, Peck KK, et al. Blood oxygen level dependent functional magnetic resonance imaging for presurgical planning. Neuroimaging Clin N Am 2014;24(4):557–71.
3. Brennan NP, Peck Kk, Holodny A. Language Mapping Using fMRI and Direct Cortical Stimulation for Brain Tumor Surgery: The Good, the Bad, and the Questionable. Top Magn Reson Imaging 2016;25: 1–10.
4. Mowinckel AM, Espeseth T, Westlye LT. Network-specific effects of age and in-scanner subject motion: a resting-state fMRI study of 238 healthy adults. Neuroimage 2012;63(3):1364–73.
5. Huettel SA, Singerman JD, McCarthy G. The effects of aging upon the hemodynamic response measured by functional MRI. Neuroimage 2001; 13(1):161–75.
6. West KL, Zuppichini MD, Turner MP, et al. BOLD hemodynamic response function changes significantly with healthy aging. Neuroimage 2019;188:198–207.
7. Morsheddost H, Asemani D, Alizadoh Shalchy M. Evaluation of Hemodynamic Response Function in

Vision and Motor Brain Regions for the Young and Elderly Adults. Basic Clin Neurosci 2015;6(1):58–68.

8. Gauthier CJ, Madjar C, Desjardins-Crépeau L, et al. Age dependence of hemodynamic response characteristics in human functional magnetic resonance imaging. Neurobiol Aging 2013;34(5):1469–85.

9. Fabiani M, Gordon BA, Maclin EL, et al. Neurovascular coupling in normal aging: a combined optical, ERP and fMRI study. Neuroimage 2014;85: 592–607. Pt 1(0 1).

10. Chen CM, Hou BL, Holodny AI. Effect of age and tumor grade on BOLD functional MR imaging in preoperative assessment of patients with glioma. Radiology 2008;248(3):971–8.

11. Yerys BE, Jankowski KF, Shook D, et al. The fMRI success rate of children and adolescents: typical development, epilepsy, attention deficit/hyperactivity disorder, and autism spectrum disorders. Hum Brain Mapp 2009;30(10):3426–35.

12. Rajagopal A, Byars A, Schapiro M, et al. Success rates for functional MR imaging in children. AJNR Am J Neuroradiol 2014;35(12):2319–25.

13. Satterthwaite TD, Wolf DH, Loughead J, et al. Impact of in-scanner head motion on multiple measures of functional connectivity: relevance for studies of neurodevelopment in youth. Neuroimage 2012;60(1): 623–32.

14. Springer JA, Binder JR, Hammeke TA, et al. Language dominance in neurologically normal and epilepsy subjects: a functional MRI study. Brain 1999; 122(Pt 11):2033–46.

15. Knecht S, Dräger B, Deppe M, et al. Handedness and hemispheric language dominance in healthy humans. Brain 2000;123(12):2512–8.

16. Bethmann A, Tempelmann C, De Bleser R, et al. Determining language laterality by fMRI and dichotic listening. Brain Res 2007;1133(1):145–57.

17. Khedr EM, Hamed E, Said A, et al. Handedness and language cerebral lateralization. Eur J Appl Physiol 2002;87(4–5):469–73.

18. Somers M, Aukes MF, Ophoff RA, et al. On the relationship between degree of hand-preference and degree of language lateralization. Brain Lang 2015;144:10–5.

19. Isaacs KL, Barr WB, Nelson PK, et al. Degree of handedness and cerebral dominance. Neurology 2006;66(12):1855–8.

20. Oldfield RC. The assessment and analysis of handedness: The Edinburgh inventory. Neuropsychologia 1971;9(1):97–113.

21. Porac C. Attempts to switch the writing hand: relationships to age and side of hand preference. Laterality 1996;1(1):35–44.

22. Siebner HR, Limmer C, Peinemann A, et al. Long-term consequences of switching handedness: a positron emission tomography study on handwriting in "converted" left-handers. J Neurosci 2002;22(7):2816–25.

23. Bogomolny DL, Petrovich NM, Hou BL, et al. Functional MRI in the brain tumor patient. Top Magn Reson Imaging 2004;15(5):325–35.

24. Belyaev AS, Peck KK, Brennan NM, et al. Clinical applications of functional MR imaging. Magn Reson Imaging Clin N Am 2013;21(2):269–78.

25. Holodny AI, Shevzov-Zebrun N, Brennan N, et al. Motor and Sensory Mapping. Neurosurg Clin 2011; 22(2):207–18.

26. Brennan N. Preparing the patient for the fMRI study and optimization of paradigm selection and delivery. In: Holodny A, editor. Functional Neuroimaging: A Clinical Approach. Informa Healthcare; 2008. p. 13–21.

27. Peck KK, Holodny AI. fMRI Clinical Applications. In: Reiser MF, Semmler W, Hricak H, editors. Magnetic resonance tomography. Berlin (Germany): Springer Science & Business Media; 2007. p. 1308–31.

28. Holodny AI, Schulder M, Liu WC, et al. Decreased BOLD functional MR activation of the motor and sensory cortices adjacent to a glioblastoma multiforme: implications for image-guided neurosurgery. AJNR Am J Neuroradiol 1999;20(4):609–12.

29. Holodny AI, Schulder M, Liu WC, et al. The effect of brain tumors on BOLD functional MR imaging activation in the adjacent motor cortex: implications for image-guided neurosurgery. AJNR Am J Neuroradiol 2000;21(8):1415–22.

30. Peck KK, Bradbury M, Petrovich N, et al. Presurgical Evaluation of Language Using Functional Magnetic Resonance Imaging in Brain Tumor Patients with Previous Surgery. Neurosurgery 2009;64(4): 644–52.

31. Fraga de Abreu VH, Peck KK, Petrovich-Brennan NM, et al. Brain Tumors: The Influence of Tumor Type and Routine MR Imaging Characteristics at BOLD Functional MR Imaging in the Primary Motor Gyrus. Radiology 2016;281:876–83.

32. Petrovich NM, Holodny AI, Brennan CW, et al. Isolated translocation of Wernicke's area to the right hemisphere in a 62-year-man with a temporoparietal glioma. AJNR Am J Neuroradiol 2004; 25(1):130–3.

33. Li Q, Dong JW, Del Ferraro G, et al. Functional Translocation of Broca's Area in a Low-Grade Left Frontal Glioma: Graph Theory Reveals the Novel, Adaptive Network Connectivity. Front Neurol 2019;10:702.

34. Fisicaro RA, Jost E, Shaw K, et al. Cortical Plasticity in the Setting of Brain Tumors. Top Magn Reson Imaging 2016;25(1):25–30.

35. Robles SG, Gatignol P, Lehericy S, et al. Long-term brain plasticity allowing a multistage surgical approach to World Health Organization Grade II gliomas in eloquent areas. J Neurosurg 2008;109(4): 615–24.

36. Duffau H. Lessons from brain mapping in surgery for low-grade glioma: insights into associations

between tumour and brain plasticity. Lancet Neurol 2005;4(8):476–86.

37. Desmurget M, Bonnetblanc F, Duffau H. Contrasting acute and slow-growing lesions: a new door to brain plasticity. Brain 2007;130(Pt 4):898–914.

38. Thiel A, Herholz K, Koyuncu A, et al. Plasticity of language networks in patients with brain tumors: a positron emission tomography activation study. Ann Neurol 2001;50(5):620–9.

39. Holodny AI, Schulder M, Ybasco A, et al. Translocation of Broca's area to the contralateral hemisphere as the result of the growth of a left inferior frontal glioma. J Comput Assist Tomogr 2002;26(6):941–3.

40. Kaplan E, Goodglass H, Weintraub S, et al. Boston naming test. Philadelphia: Lea & Febiger; 1983.

41. de Guibert C, Maumet C, Ferre JC, et al. FMRI language mapping in children: a panel of language tasks using visual and auditory stimulation without reading or metalinguistic requirements. Neuroimage 2010;51(2):897–909.

42. Amunts K, Schleicher A, Burgel U, et al. Broca's region revisited: cytoarchitecture and intersubject variability. J Comp Neurol 1999;412(2):319–41.

43. Sanai N, Mirzadeh Z, Berger MS. Functional outcome after language mapping for glioma resection. N Engl J Med 2008;358(1):18–27.

44. Keller SS, Crow T, Foundas A, et al. Broca's area: nomenclature, anatomy, typology and asymmetry. Brain Lang 2009;109(1):29–48.

45. Mohr JP, Pessin MS, Finkelstein S, et al. Broca aphasia: pathologic and clinical. Neurology 1978;28(4):311–24.

46. Miura K, Nakamura Y, Miura F, et al. Functional magnetic resonance imaging to word generation task in a patient with Broca's aphasia. J Neurol 1999;246(10):939–42.

47. Quinones-Hinojosa A, Ojemann SG, Sanai N, et al. Preoperative correlation of intraoperative cortical mapping with magnetic resonance imaging landmarks to predict localization of the Broca area. J Neurosurg 2003;99(2):311–8.

48. Middlebrooks EH, Yagmurlu K, Szaflarski JP, et al. A contemporary framework of language processing in the human brain in the context of preoperative and intraoperative language mapping. Neuroradiology 2017;59(1):69–87.

49. Bookheimer S. Functional MRI of language: new approaches to understanding the cortical organization of semantic processing. Annu Rev Neurosci 2002; 25:151–88.

50. Binder JR. Current Controversies on Wernicke's Area and its Role in Language. Curr Neurol Neurosci Rep 2017;17(8):58.

51. Chang EF, Raygor KP, Berger MS. Contemporary model of language organization: an overview for neurosurgeons. J Neurosurg 2015;122(2):250–61.

52. Burns MS, Fahy J. Broca's area: rethinking classical concepts from a neuroscience perspective. Top Stroke Rehabil 2010;17(6):401–10.

53. Tremblay P, Dick AS. Broca and Wernicke are dead, or moving past the classic model of language neurobiology. Brain Lang 2016;162:60–71.

54. Dong JW, Brennan NM, Izzo G, et al. fMRI activation in the middle frontal gyrus as an indicator of hemispheric dominance for language in brain tumor patients: a comparison with Broca's area. Neuroradiology 2016; 58(5):513–20.

55. Pillai J. Language. In: Holodny A, editor. Functional Neuroimaging: A Clinical Approach. Informa Healthcare; 2008. p. 51–66.

56. Bathla G, Gene MN, Peck KK, et al. Resting State Functional Connectivity of the Supplementary Motor Area to Motor and Language Networks in Patients with Brain Tumors. J Neuroimaging 2019;29(4):521–6.

57. Peck KK, Bradbury M, Psaty EL, et al. Joint activation of the supplementary motor area and presupplementary motor area during simultaneous motor and language functional MRI. Neuroreport 2009; 20(5):487–91.

58. Lyo JK, Arevalo-Perez J, Petrovich Brennan N, et al. Pre-operative fMRI localization of the supplementary motor area and its relationship with postoperative speech deficits. Neuroradiol J 2015;28(3):281–8.

59. Nelson L, Lapsiwala S, Haughton VM, et al. Preoperative mapping of the supplementary motor area in patients harboring tumors in the medial frontal lobe. J Neurosurg 2002;97(5):1108–14.

60. Oh A, Duerden EG, Pang EW. The role of the insula in speech and language processing. Brain Lang 2014;135:96–103.

61. Eickhoff SB, Heim S, Zilles K, et al. A systems perspective on the effective connectivity of overt speech production. Philos Trans A Math Phys Eng Sci 2009;367(1896):2399–421.

62. Dronkers NF. A new brain region for coordinating speech articulation. Nature 1996;384(6605):159–61.

63. Ackermann H, Riecker A. The contribution(s) of the insula to speech production: a review of the clinical and functional imaging literature. Brain Struct Funct 2010;214(5–6):419–33.

64. Shafto MA, Burke DM, Stamatakis EA, et al. On the tip-of-the-tongue: neural correlates of increased word-finding failures in normal aging. J Cogn Neurosci 2007;19(12):2060–70.

65. Binder JR, Desai RH, Graves WW, et al. Where is the semantic system? A critical review and meta-analysis of 120 functional neuroimaging studies. Cereb Cortex 2009;19(12):2767–96.

66. Meyler A, Keller TA, Cherkassky VL, et al. Modifying the brain activation of poor readers during sentence comprehension with extended remedial instruction:

a longitudinal study of neuroplasticity. Neuropsychologia 2008;46(10):2580–92.

67. Meyler A, Keller TA, Cherkassky VL, et al. Brain activation during sentence comprehension among good and poor readers. Cereb Cortex 2007;17(12):2780–7.

68. Hartwigsen G, Baumgaertner A, Price CJ, et al. Phonological decisions require both the left and right supramarginal gyri. Proc Natl Acad Sci U S A 2010;107(38):16494–9.

69. Roux FE, Boetto S, Sacko O, et al. Writing, calculating, and finger recognition in the region of the angular gyrus: a cortical stimulation study of Gerstmann syndrome. J Neurosurg 2003;99(4):716–27.

70. Chang EF, Breshears JD, Raygor KP, et al. Stereotactic probability and variability of speech arrest and anomia sites during stimulation mapping of the language dominant hemisphere. J Neurosurg 2017;126(1):114–21.

71. Petrovich Brennan NM, Whalen S, de Morales Branco D, et al. Object naming is a more sensitive measure of speech localization than number counting: Converging evidence from direct cortical stimulation and fMRI. Neuroimage 2007;37(Suppl 1):S100–8.

72. Kesavadas C, Thomas B. Clinical applications of functional MRI in epilepsy. Indian J Radiol Imaging 2008;18(3):210–7.

73. Wang A, Peters TM, de Ribaupierre S, et al. Functional magnetic resonance imaging for language mapping in temporal lobe epilepsy. Epilepsy research and treatment. 2012;vol. 2012:198183. https://doi.org/10.1155/2012/198183.

74. Woermann FG, Jokeit H, Luerding R, et al. Language lateralization by Wada test and fMRI in 100 patients with epilepsy. Neurology 2003;61(5):699–701.

75. Janecek JK, Swanson SJ, Sabsevitz DS, et al. Language lateralization by fMRI and Wada testing in 229 patients with epilepsy: rates and predictors of discordance. Epilepsia 2013;54(2):314–22.

76. Gutbrod K, Spring D, Degonda N, et al. Determination of language dominance: Wada test and fMRI compared using a novel sentence task. J Neuroimaging 2012;22(3):266–74.

77. Rosenberg K, Nossek E, Liebling R, et al. Prediction of neurological deficits and recovery after surgery in the supplementary motor area: a prospective study in 26 patients. J Neurosurg 2010;113(6):1152–63.

78. Kocak M, Ulmer JL, Sahin Ugurel M, et al. Motor homunculus: passive mapping in healthy volunteers by using functional MR imaging–initial results. Radiology 2009;251(2):485–92.

Methods of Analysis
Functional MRI for Presurgical Planning

Kyung K. Peck, PhD[a,b,*], Nicholas S. Cho, BA[c], Andrei I. Holodny, MD[d]

KEY WORDS

- Functional MRI (fMRI) • Methods of analysis • Pre-processing • Post-processing
- Statistical analysis

KEY POINTS

- Task instruction and rehearsal are the most important steps during an fMRI procedure.
- Data processing steps must be taken to optimize the signal that is associated with specific functional tasks and to minimize any noise-related signal.
- Pre-processed data significantly affects statistical analysis, which has a great impact on image interpretation.
- Algorithms for head motion detection and correction, the theory and practicalities associated with data processing remain complex and constantly evolving.

INTRODUCTION

Since its discovery in the early 1990s, functional MRI (fMRI) has been used to study brain function and to advance clinical care.[1,2] One well-established application of fMRI in the clinical setting is in neurosurgical mapping for patients with brain tumors near eloquent cortical areas.[3–5] The main goal of neurosurgery is to maximize tumor resection while sparing important brain structures near the tumor, which relies on the proper identification of eloquent cortical areas.[6–9] However, interestingly, there is considerable anatomic variation in the human brain between individuals, and the presence of a tumor can lead to cortical plasticity that recruits cerebral areas for tasks that are not originally associated with that region.[10–13] As a result, the location of eloquent cortical areas adjacent to a tumor cannot be accurately defined by simply examining a structural brain image. In addition, one must be careful to acknowledge the existence of neurovascular uncoupling (NVU) that may also influence the blood-oxygen-level-dependent (BOLD) fMRI signal and can lead to false negative results (see separate article elsewhere in this issue).[14–19] The goal of clinical fMRI is to preoperatively identify important functional areas associated with specific functional tasks critical in the patients' daily life, such as hand movement and language function.[18,20,21] For example, when a lesion presents in the vicinity of important areas like sensory motor or language areas, surgeons may request an fMRI scan to know how close the regions of activation are located near the lesion to best plan the

Funding information: National Institutes of Health (NIH): NIH-NIGMS Training Grant GM008042 (N.S. Cho), NIH-NIBIB R01 EB022720 (Makse and Holodny, principal investigators (PIs)), NIH-NCI R21 CA220144 (A.I. Holodny and K.K. Peck, PI's), NIH-NCI U54 CA137788 (Ahles, PI), NIH-NCI P30 CA008748 (Thompson, PI).

[a] Department of Medical Physics, Memorial Sloan Kettering Cancer Center, 1275 York Avenue, New York, NY 10021, USA; [b] Department of Radiology, Memorial Sloan Kettering Cancer Center, 1275 York Avenue, New York, NY 10021, USA; [c] Medical Scientist Training Program, David Geffen School of Medicine at UCLA, 885 Tiverton Drive, Los Angeles, CA 90024, USA; [d] Department of Radiology, Memorial Sloan Kettering Cancer Center, 1275 York Avenue, New York, NY 10065, USA
* Corresponding author. Department of Medical Physics, Memorial Sloan Kettering Cancer Center, 1275 York Avenue, New York, NY 10021.
E-mail address: peckk@mskcc.org

Neuroimag Clin N Am 31 (2021) 23–32
https://doi.org/10.1016/j.nic.2020.09.006

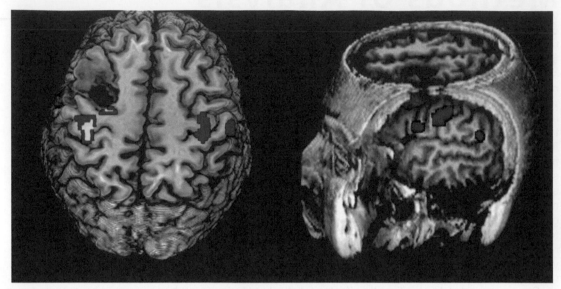

Fig. 1. Examples of presurgical functional MRI scans in a 3D rendering map for a patient with a tumor in the left hemisphere. (*A*) During a hand motor task, activation in the precentral gyrus is posterior to the lesion. (*B*) During a language task, activation in Broca's and Wernicke's areas is inferior to the lesion.

surgery, including for intraoperative brain mapping or awake brain surgery (Fig. 1).

WORKFLOW IN CLINICAL FUNCTIONAL MRI
General Workflow

To obtain successful fMRI maps for presurgical planning, there are several important steps involved. The following diagram shows the typical workflow for a clinical fMRI procedure (Fig. 2).

First, the neurosurgeon refers the patient to the fMRI team. The presence of any neurologic deficits should be noted to help guide the fMRI team with the lesion location. The fMRI team will also determine the lesion location by examining any previous images of the patients' lesion, if available, and

Presurgical planning fMRI schema

Surgeon refers patient and gives brief history of neurological deficit, if any
↓
Review images for lesion location
↓
Choose fMRI paradigm targeted to lesion location
↓
Test patient on fMRI paradigms prior to scanning
↓
Acquiring fMRI dataset
↓
Data Processing and Analysis
↓
Prepare Report

Fig. 2. Presurgical planning fMRI schema.

account for its potential growth or spread. Based on the lesion location, specific fMRI paradigms are prescribed to elucidate the nearby and/or affected cortical areas via task function.

On the day of the scan, the fMRI team begins by instructing the patient regarding the functional tasks that the patient will perform in the scanner. During the scan itself, the patient's performance is monitored using the available real-time pre-processing software in the MRI suite. Current modern scanners incorporate some capability to perform *t*-test or Z-score analysis on a voxel-by-voxel level in real-time. This quick, real-time review of the fMRI activation will allow the fMRI team to have knowledge about the quality of the data acquisition, guiding the team to either continue with the scan or to re-conduct the scan. The completed fMRI and anatomic dataset can then be transferred to an off-line computer for pre-processing and statistical analysis. A neuroradiologist then reviews the functional activation maps generated, and a report is written for the neurosurgeon.

Task Instruction and Monitoring the Task Performance

The importance of following 2 procedures before any scanning is conducted cannot be overstated: *task instruction* and *monitoring task performance*. In clinical fMRI, the patient's task instruction and rehearsal before the scan are of utmost importance and more critical than the image processing itself. The success of a fMRI scan also mainly depends on the subject's task performance: even if you have the highest quality MRI scanner, you cannot generate a good fMRI scan if the subject's task performance is poor. Task performance is especially important when the scan is used for pre-surgical planning because the patients may have neurologic deficits related to their lesion.

The subject's task performance is also directly related to how well the subject understood the task instruction. Before a subject is scanned, a fMRI specialist instructs the subject about the functional tasks that will be performed in the scanner. During this procedure, the specialist should be able to gauge the subject's performance level as they rehearse the task before going to the scanner. For example, hand or foot weakness can be evaluated when rehearsing motor tasks. If the subject shows very weak hand or foot motor strength, the fMRI specialist may need to make a decision to change the paradigm from a self-controlled task to an externally controlled stimulation for sensory motor task. For language function, several assessments including the Boston Naming Test can be performed to assess for any language deficits. If the subject has a language deficit, then it would be better to apply several different types of language paradigms because one language paradigm could be easier than another for the subject, and different paradigms may elicit different brain activations that can be interpreted together as a whole for general language function. Careful paradigm selection according to the patient's condition, proper instruction, and practice of the paradigms prior to scanning also reduces difficulties with head motion artifacts and poor or inconsistent task performance. These nontechnical considerations during an fMRI scan can often be overlooked, but they remain vital for a successful clinical fMRI scan.

IMAGE PRE-PROCESSING
Purpose of Functional MRI Data Processing

After acquiring the fMRI data, fMRI data processing is conducted to maximize the signal and filter out the noise that is associated with the task performance (Fig. 3). This process involves reducing the artifactual signal in the voxel time course that is, not part of the subject's functional task performance. When this process is finished, there is improved detectability of statistically significant activation clusters that can be used to generate functional maps for presurgical scanning. fMRI data processing is generally conducted through several, essential steps including image quality assessment, head motion correction, spatial smoothing, and linear trend removal.

Normally, the fMRI data is processed using commercial or freely downloadable software (eg, FSL and AFNI[22,23]). Commercial software is designed to be user-friendly and provides automatic or manual pre-processing tools. However, the fMRI data obtained from patients occasionally needs more complicated and patient-specific image processing steps that cannot be handled by the pre-determined automated processes found in commercial software. Therefore, additional advanced software may be used to tackle complicated issues including randomly-occurring artifactual images, severe head motion, and incorrect task performance.

Image Quality Assessment

After the raw fMRI data are transferred for data processing, it is essential to carefully review the images and time courses, especially the areas where activation is expected. Any sources of artifacts and noise-related abrupt signal change in the data should be identified and removed or minimized. Performing these image quality checks consistently throughout the pre-processing steps significantly improves the final images used for clinical interpretation.

Functional MRI Artifacts

The main artifacts in fMRI are caused by susceptibility, which are due to local magnetic field inhomogeneity. Common sources of these artifacts are at air-tissue interfaces such as the ear and nasal canals, which can cause signal loss in the auditory cortex and frontal lobe, respectively. There are other potential sources of susceptibility artifacts including the sphenoid sinus in the inferior frontal cortex and geometric distortion due to scanner Bo field inhomogeneity. There are also subject-related artifacts including those caused by the movement of brain parenchyma and the subject's motion due to heart rate, respiratory rate, and bulk head motion. Cardiac pulsation artifacts can appear as large as a few percent signal change of BOLD contrast. Bulk head motion can cause voxels on the periphery of the brain to appear activated.[24-26] Reviewing the images in "real-time mode" and checking temporal variations in the time series often allows for identifying problematic volumes or slices that should be removed before further processing steps (Fig. 4).

Head Motion

Motion is a major problem for fMRI studies, for it is the greatest cause of fMRI examination failure. In

Pre-processing stream for fMRI data

Image Reconstruction
↓
Check Image Quality
↓
Motion Correction
↓
Spatial Smoothing
↓
Statistical Analysis

Fig. 3. Pre-processing stream for fMRI data.

clinical fMRI, patients tend to show more frequent unintended head and body movements due to their underlying, neurologic condition than healthy control subjects. Motion is also more easily prevented than corrected. Therefore, patients must be specifically instructed how head motion can degrade the image quality and may lead to a repeated scan. In the scanner, ensuring maximal patient comfort can decrease the chance of motion. In addition, vocal feedback and encouragement right before each scan will help to minimize motion artifacts.

As task-related BOLD signal percentage changes are small (on the order of single-digit percentage changes) and because data analysis is based on signal variation in the voxel time series, even small head motion can heavily confound statistical analyses.[27] Motion can occur during different paradigms and in different directions; leg motion for foot motor tasks can cause head movement in the inferior-to-superior direction, while the tongue motor task cause shifts in head placement.

Motion during fMRI can be of 2 kinds: *randomly timed motion* or *stimulus-correlated motion*. Randomly timed motion (that is not correlated with the stimulus task) can block real activity by increasing false negatives in the activation map. False negatives may increase when the random motion occurs during the baseline volumes where no task-induced activation should be present. On the other hand, stimulus-correlated motion creates false positives, as voxels of higher signal intensity can be shifted into surrounding areas of the activating region that are originally occupied by other voxels of lower signal intensity. If 2 neighboring voxels differ in intrinsic brightness by 15%, then a motion of 10% of a voxel dimension can result in a 1.5% signal change which is comparable to the BOLD signal percent change during stimulus activation at 1.5 T.[25] Stimulus-correlated motion is particularly problematic because most software programs do not have a tool to separate true activity from activation due to head motion.[26] Stimulus-correlated motion can be especially severe in areas lying near the high-contrast boundaries in the brain (**Fig. 5**). Percent signal change of the voxels due to stimulus-correlated motion is typically much higher than that of the true activated voxels. The percent signal change could be used as a threshold to remove such false positive voxels.

Motion Correction

Despite efforts to minimize motion, head motion can still occur and must be corrected during processing. During motion correction processing, we are assuming that the same voxel represents the same location in the brain throughout the scans and the signal change in the same voxel between volumes is mainly due to activation coupling with task performance. Many motion correction

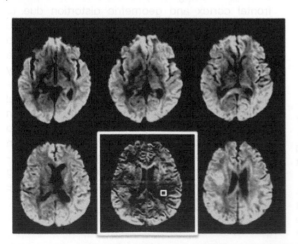
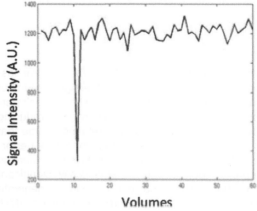

Fig. 4. Artifactual image shown in the white outline and the associated abnormal signal fluctuation in the time course in the region of interest.

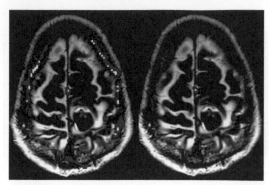

Fig. 5. Artifactual activation from stimulus-correlated motion.

algorithms and software packages typically are applied during pre-processing before statistical analysis, with no single package producing dramatically better results than others.[27] Following each motion correction step, the fMRI data can be quality control checked by looking at the motion parameter plots and viewing the images in "cine mode" to check whether the mismatch between slices has improved.

Generally, correction using rigid body motion (ie, no change in the size or shape) by estimating 3-dimensional (3D) motion parameters (the set of 3 translocation and 3 rotation parameters) is used to minimize the difference between the reference volume and the other volumes. Usually, one can choose the reference volume at the initial volumes of the scan, and then register all remaining volumes against the reference volume. This is because if 2D functional matching anatomic images are acquired before functional scan, then presumably, the initial functional volumes would be matched the most with the 2D anatomic images. Next, the sum of absolute intensity differences between voxels in the reference volumes and the other volumes is calculated. The 6 motion parameters mentioned previously can be used to detrend the data against correlation with the movements as a to minimize motion-correlated false positive activation.[28] However, this approach should be used with a caution because it can cause increased false negative voxels if the averaged time course associated with stimulus-correlated motion is similar to the time course associated with task-induced activation.

Three-dimensional volume registration is generally useful for intra- and intersession alignment. However, this approach cannot correct motions that occur within the time equal to or less than the repetition time (TR) since this approach assumes a rigid movement of the entire volume. This limitation of being unable to correct for motion that occurs

for a time shorter than the length of the TR emphasizes the importance of having the patient hold as still as possible. If such significant motion occurs in one of stimulus blocks, it would be better to exclude the volume in the following processing steps.

Spatial Smoothing

Generally, in fMRI data, high spatial frequencies likely represent noise components whereas low frequencies are changes produced by blood flow and thus are more likely to represent the BOLD signal due to neurovascular coupling (NVC). Spatial smoothing increases the signal-to-noise ratio (SNR) by suppressing high frequency noise components and enhancing low frequency signals. This is a helpful technique to use in data processing because it enhances the likelihood of determining eloquent cortices in the brain during functional tasks. By suppressing high frequencies, smoothing increases the area of the brain where small signal changes from NVC can be detected,[29] thus allowing clinical decisions for a patient to be made from optimized functional information.

In spatial smoothing, voxels are averaged with their surrounding neighbors in an image, which causes the blurring of sharp edges. Smoothing is performed by convolving the image with a point spread function using a Gaussian kernel with a width between 4 to 8 mm full width half maximum (FWHM). The FWHM provides an estimation of smoothing of a Gaussian kernel as the standard deviation(s) is calculated using the relation $s = FWHM \times 0.425$. After convolving with a point spread function, a matrix of the same size is created. Then, the image is convolved with the matrix. By performing these steps, the signal from each voxel spreads out to surrounding voxels. The optimal width of the smoothing filter determines the extent of blurring and is chosen to closely match the size of the region activated.[30] A general rule of thumb for fMRI data is choosing an FWHM twice the voxel size. For example, if FOV = 240 mm and 64×64 matrix with in-plane resolution = 3.75×3.75 mm, the FWHM should be approximately 6 to 8 mm. As FWHM increases, there is a tradeoff between better activation maps through increased SNR and increased image blurring, as shown in **Fig. 6**.

Before smoothing, it is important to note the task involved and the expected area of localization during imaging. Signal changes produced during language and cognitive tasks are smaller than in motor-sensory tasks. For example, BOLD responses in the motor-sensory system are generally large ($\sim$2%–6%), robust, and within a narrow area of possible activation (a few millimeters across). Thus, in presurgical mapping of the

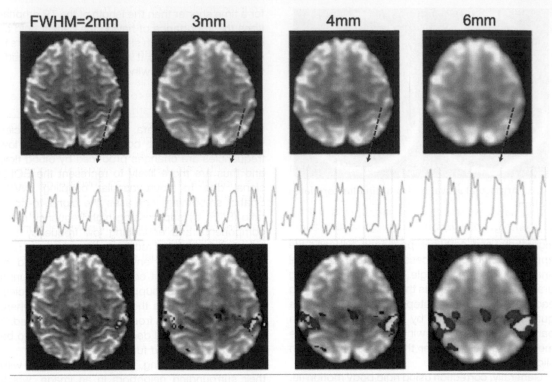

Fig. 6. The effect of different size of Gaussian kernel applied to an image with in-plane resolution 2 × 2 mm. A region of interest (*red arrow*) is placed in a hand motor gyrus and the associated time course is displayed. Reduced high-frequency noise is obtained with increased kernel size.

motor cortex using fMRI, it is better to use narrow or sometimes even no smoothing because an accurate and robust activation map can often be produced. However, during language tasks, BOLD responses are much less (~1%–3% signal change) in Broca's and Wernicke's Areas. To detect these smaller signal changes, a larger kernel size for spatial smoothing is recommended. A larger kernel size increases the SNR, thereby increasing the likelihood of retaining voxels responding to functional tasks.

Linear Trend Removal

Another frequently observed issue is a near-linear baseline signal drift (0.0–0.015 Hz). This temporal drift shows a linear trend and is likely due to scanner instabilities causing changes in the local magnetic field. The low frequency signal drift issue affects statistical analysis and power by altering the volume of activation.[31] Because the drifts are slowly rising and falling, the drifts can be effectively removed by using a high-pass filter. Several methods exist to remove the drift from analysis such as linear models, low-order polynomial models, and spline models.[25,27,28,32]

STATISTICAL ANALYSIS

For statistical analysis, a hypothesis-driven statistical analysis is usually used to identify areas showing increased response as compared with baseline conditions. For example, the *t*-test can compare 2 conditions (for example, stimulus-off period and on period) and test if there is a mean difference. The analysis of variance test, as an extension of *t*-test, deals with more than 2 conditions. Generally, language and other cognitive tasks produce activations that are widely distributed with less percentage signal change, which makes the *t*-test approach not generally adequate.

Analysis Methods: Correlation Analysis

The cross-correlation test is the most popular analysis method in clinical fMRI because the method addresses the changing time courses between stimulus-on and off periods (**Fig. 7**). For cross-correlation analysis, a boxcar reference waveform is built, representing the stimulus-on and off periods. When the patient is performing a rest state and a task, a value of 0 and 1, respectively, are set. The cross-correlation analysis

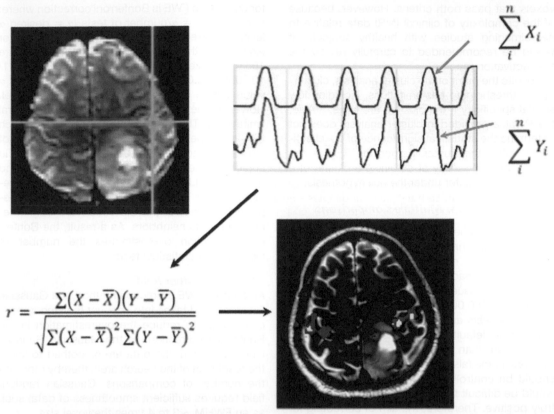

Fig. 7. Cross-correlation analysis. The green crosshairs show a voxel in the hand motor area. The voxel's corresponding time course is shown in black. The waveform convolved with hemodynamic response based on the block paradigm is shown in red. The waveform correlates with BOLD signal across each voxel.

produces 2 results for each voxel. One is the magnitude of signal change and the other is statistical significance of the magnitude calculated (correlation and the corresponding *P* value, respectively).

If a patient's task performance shows delayed responses, there are 2 methods to address the issue with correlation analysis. If the delay occurs consistently, then the designed ideal function can be shifted to match the delay. If the delay occurs inconsistently, then the hemodynamic response in the expected area can be used as an ideal function in the method. In this method, motion parameters saved during head motion correction can be used as a regressor, and any voxels that are highly correlated with the motion profile should be removed. Motion-induced false positive activations can be minimized in this way.

Setting up a threshold
Corrected *P*<.01 remains the gold standard for general neuroimaging analysis, but setting a uniform statistical threshold in clinical fMRI is not

always straightforward because in many situations, data quality often varies between patients scanned. If our criteria are too conservative (ie, if our *P* value is too low), the power to detect meaningful results will be low, and Type II errors (false negative) will increase. If our criteria are too liberal (if *P* value is too high), the result will become contaminated by Type I errors (false positives). Ideally, the goal of setting a threshold is to maximize the number of true positives while minimizing false positives.

Cluster analysis
Another method to remove artifactually activated voxels is cluster analysis. In cluster analysis, a minimum statistical volume of a group of contiguous voxels, or a cluster, is set so that only the significant clusters larger than the minimum volume are visualized. Cluster analysis typically has good sensitivity, but there is a risk to miss small but significant voxels because the cluster threshold is based on the voxel size. Therefore, thresholds using both voxel level inference and cluster level inference should be properly applied to identify

voxels that pass both criteria. However, because of the complexity of clinical fMRI data relative to neuroimaging studies with healthy subjects, it would be recommended to carefully review the final activation map.

Despite the merit of the cluster analysis, cluster-based thresholding has limitations, including low spatial specificity if the clusters are large.[33] Also, the P value provided in cluster analysis does not determine the statistical significance of voxel activation within the cluster. Rather, the P value describes the probability of obtaining a cluster of a given size or greater under the null hypothesis.

Analysis Methods: Multiple Comparisons

An important issue in fMRI data analysis is setting an appropriate threshold for statistical activation maps. However, running the statistical analyses separately for each voxel leads to the multiple comparisons issue. For instance, if the brain is divided into 100,000 voxels, then that means that voxel-level tests are repeated more than 100,000 times. If the default P value threshold, $P<.01$, there will be more than 1000 false positive voxels.[34,35] As a result, the false positive rate across all voxels should be controlled and reduced. Otherwise, it would be difficult to know if an activation result is truly positive. Therefore, the aim of correcting for multiple comparisons is to identify areas of activity that reflect true effects. In the actual clinical setting, it is challenging to find an appropriate balance between trying to minimize false positives (Type I error) while not being too omitting true effects (Type II error). If the region(s) interested are known, the analysis can be limited to just those voxels with a prior hypothesis. In this way, the number of voxels can be reduced and the multiple comparison that should be corrected can be reduced.

Software used to analyze fMRI data can use various methods for multiple comparisons correction. For example, there is the Family-Wise Error (FWE) correction that is based on the Bonferroni correction or the Random Field Theory method. The False Discovery Rate (FDR) correction method has also been used to control for multiple comparisons.[36] Image software tools automatically calculate the corrected threshold while analyzing the fMRI files based on the number of tested voxels and the number of voxels reporting significant activity before correction.

Family-wise error
FWE is the probability of finding one or more false positives among all hypothesis tests. If FWE = 0.01, the probability of finding one or more false positives is 1%. The simplest method

for controlling FWE is Bonferroni correction where: α (corrected) = α/number of tests |α = desired α level |α (corrected) = FEW-corrected α level. For example, if the desired α = 0.01 and there are 100,000 voxels to test, α (corrected) = 0.01/100,000 = 0.0000001. Therefore, the corrected α value will be much lower than the desired level. However, the Bonferroni correction has several limitations. The correction assumes that each test is independent, but in reality, voxels are not completely independent because time courses in adjacent voxels tend to be highly correlated and because BOLD activity itself often spans large regions. Also, spatial smoothing during preprocessing means that no voxels are truly independent of its neighbors. As a result, the Bonferroni correction overestimates the number of independent statistical tests.

Gaussian random field
As another FWE correction method, the Gaussian Random Field takes into account the smoothness of the data to reduce the overestimation in the Bonferroni correction. In the Gaussian Random Field correction, the data are smoothed to lower the resolution of the search area, thereby reducing the number of comparisons. Gaussian random field requires sufficient smoothness of data, such as an FWHM ~3 to 4 times the voxel size.

False discovery rate
The FWE mentioned previously ensures that false positives will be controlled per all hypothesis tests. For example, α (FWE-corrected) = 0.01 (1%) of contrast (across all voxels) will have a single false positive. In FDR, it controls the number of false positives within the significant results obtained from a family of tests. If α (FDR-corrected = 0.01), 1% of active voxels will be false positives. That means the FDR will get more true active voxels, but as a downside, it will have some false positive voxels.

SUMMARY

There are many technical and nontechnical steps involved in a successful clinical fMRI scan. The output from scanning and analysis can only be as good as the input, so task instruction and rehearsal are the most important steps during an fMRI procedure. After fMRI data acquisition, proper data processing steps must be taken to optimize the signal that is associated with specific functional tasks and to minimize any noise-related signal. Properly pre-processed data significantly affects statistical analysis, which has a great impact on image interpretation. Even though there is general agreement on how to process clinical fMRI data, such as algorithms for head motion detection and correction, the theory and practicalities associated with data processing remain complex and constantly evolving.

DISCLOSURE

K.K. Peck and N.S. Cho have nothing to disclose. AH is the Owner/President of fMRI Consultants, LLC, a purely educational entity.

REFERENCES

1. Belyaev AS, Peck KK, Brennan NM, et al. Clinical applications of functional MR imaging. Magn Reson Imaging Clin N Am 2013;21:269–78.
2. Holodny AI, Shevzov-Zebrun N, Brennan N, et al. Motor and sensory mapping. Neurosurg Clin N Am 2011;22:207–18, viii.
3. Gabriel M, Brennan NP, Peck KK, et al. Blood oxygen level dependent functional magnetic resonance imaging for presurgical planning. Neuroimaging Clin N Am 2014;24:557–71.
4. Jacobs AH, Kracht LW, Gossmann A, et al. Imaging in neurooncology. NeuroRx 2005;2:333–47.
5. Petrella JR, Shah LM, Harris KM, et al. Preoperative functional MR imaging localization of language and motor areas: effect on therapeutic decision making in patients with potentially resectable brain tumors. Radiology 2006;240:793–802.
6. Brennan NP, Peck KK, Holodny A. Language mapping using fMRI and direct cortical stimulation for brain tumor surgery: the good, the bad, and the questionable. Top Magn Reson Imaging 2016;25: 1–10.
7. Gupta A, Shah A, Young RJ, et al. Imaging of brain tumors: functional magnetic resonance imaging and diffusion tensor imaging. Neuroimaging Clin N Am 2010;20:379–400.
8. Holodny AI, Nusbaum AO, Festa S, et al. Correlation between the degree of contrast enhancement and the volume of peritumoral edema in meningiomas and malignant gliomas. Neuroradiology 1999;41: 820–5.
9. Pan C, Peck KK, Young RJ, et al. Somatotopic organization of motor pathways in the internal capsule: a probabilistic diffusion tractography study. AJNR Am J Neuroradiol 2012;33:1274–80.
10. Fisicaro RA, Jost E, Shaw K, et al. Cortical plasticity in the setting of brain tumors. Top Magn Reson Imaging 2016;25:25–30.
11. Holodny AI, Schulder M, Ybasco A, et al. Translocation of Broca's area to the contralateral hemisphere as the result of the growth of a left inferior frontal glioma. J Comput Assist Tomogr 2002;26:941–3.
12. Li Q, Dong JW, Del Ferraro G, et al. Functional translocation of Broca's area in a low-grade left frontal glioma: graph theory reveals the novel, adaptive network connectivity. Front Neurol 2019;10:702.
13. Petrovich NM, Holodny AI, Brennan CW, et al. Isolated translocation of Wernicke's area to the right hemisphere in a 62-year-man with a temporoparietal glioma. AJNR Am J Neuroradiol 2004;25: 130–3.
14. Chen CM, Hou BL, Holodny AI. Effect of age and tumor grade on BOLD functional MR imaging in preoperative assessment of patients with glioma. Radiology 2008;248:971–8.
15. Del Ferraro G, Moreno A, Min B, et al. Finding influential nodes for integration in brain networks using optimal percolation theory. Nat Commun 2018;9: 2274.
16. Fraga de Abreu VH, Peck KK, Petrovich-Brennan NM, et al. Brain tumors: the influence of tumor type and routine mr imaging characteristics at BOLD Functional MR Imaging in the Primary Motor Gyrus. Radiology 2016;281:876–83.
17. Mallela AN, Peck KK, Petrovich-Brennan NM, et al. Altered resting-state functional connectivity in the hand motor network in glioma patients. Brain Connect 2016;6:587–95.
18. Peck KK, Bradbury M, Petrovich N, et al. Presurgical evaluation of language using functional magnetic resonance imaging in brain tumor patients with previous surgery. Neurosurgery 2009;64:644–52 [discussion: 652–3].
19. Sun H, Vachha B, Laino ME, et al. Decreased hand motor resting-state functional connectivity in patients with glioma: analysis of factors including neurovascular uncoupling. Radiology 2020;294: 610–21.
20. Kim MJ, Holodny AI, Hou BL, et al. The effect of prior surgery on blood oxygen level-dependent functional MR imaging in the preoperative assessment of brain tumors. AJNR Am J Neuroradiol 2005;26:1980–5.
21. Li Q, Del Ferraro G, Pasquini L, et al. Core language brain network for fMRI language task used in clinical applications. Netw Neurosci 2020;4:134–54.
22. Cox RW. AFNI: software for analysis and visualization of functional magnetic resonance neuroimages. Comput Biomed Res 1996;29:162–73.
23. Woolrich MW, Jbabdi S, Patenaude B, et al. Bayesian analysis of neuroimaging data in FSL. Neuroimage 2009;45:S173–86.
24. Dagli MS, Ingeholm JE, Haxby JV. Localization of cardiac-induced signal change in fMRI. Neuroimage 1999;9:407–15.
25. Frank LR, Buxton RB, Wong EC. Estimation of respiration-induced noise fluctuations from under-sampled multislice fMRI data. Magn Reson Med 2001;45:635–44.
26. Thacker NA, Burton E, Lacey AJ, et al. The effects of motion on parametric fMRI analysis techniques. Physiol Meas 1999;20:251–63.

27. Friston KJ, Ashburner J, Frith CD, et al. Spatial registration and normalization of images. Hum Brain Mapp 1995;3:165–89.

28. Jiang A, Kennedy DN, Baker JR, et al. Motion detection and correction in functional MR imaging. Hum Brain Mapp 1995;3:224–35.

29. Parrish TB, Gitelman DR, LaBar KS, et al. Impact of signal-to-noise on functional MRI. Magn Reson Med 2000;44:925–32.

30. Friston KJ, Holmes AP, Poline JB, et al. Analysis of fMRI time-series revisited. Neuroimage 1995;2:45–53.

31. Friston KJ, Williams S, Howard R, et al. Movement-related effects in fMRI time-series. Magn Reson Med 1996;35:346–55.

32. Hajnal JV, Myers R, Oatridge A, et al. Artifacts due to stimulus correlated motion in functional imaging of the brain. Magn Reson Med 1994;31:283–91.

33. Woo C-W, Krishnan A, Wager TD. Cluster-extent based thresholding in fMRI analyses: pitfalls and recommendations. NeuroImage 2014;91:412–9.

34. Bennett CM, Miller MB, Wolford GL. Neural correlates of interspecies perspective taking in the post-mortem Atlantic Salmon: an argument for multiple comparisons correction. NeuroImage 2009;47: S125.

35. Nichols T, Hayasaka S. Controlling the familywise error rate in functional neuroimaging: a comparative review. Stat Methods Med Res 2003;12:419–46.

36. Genovese CR, Lazar NA, Nichols T. Thresholding of statistical maps in functional neuroimaging using the false discovery rate. Neuroimage 2002;15: 870–8.

Functional Brain Anatomy

Raquel A. Moreno, MD[a,b,*], Andrei I. Holodny, MD[a]

KEYWORDS

- fMR imaging • Eloquent cortex • Broca's area • Wernicke's area
- Supplementary motor area (SMA) • Primary motor cortex

KEY POINTS

- Knowledge of functional neuroanatomy is essential to design the most appropriate clinical fMR imaging paradigms and to properly interpret fMR imaging study results.
- The correlation between neuroanatomy and brain function is also very useful in general radiologic practice, as it improves the radiologist's ability to read routine brain examinations.
- Functional MR imaging is used primarily to determine the areas involved in functioning of movements, speech, and vision, which are of the greatest interest in presurgical studies.
- Preoperative fMR imaging findings also play a key role in the neurosurgeon's decision to perform a biopsy, a subtotal resection, or a maximal resection using awake craniotomy.

INTRODUCTION

Knowledge of functional neuroanatomy is essential to design the most appropriate clinical functional MR imaging (fMR imaging) paradigms and to properly interpret fMR imaging study results. This article reviews the foundations of brain anatomy by discussing the functional areas of the brain, focusing on the regions involved in movement, language, and vision, which are of the greatest interest in presurgical studies.[1]

The correlation between neuroanatomy and brain function is also very useful in general radiologic practice, as it improves the radiologist's ability to read routine brain examinations. Research has demonstrated that experience in fMR imaging improves accurate identification of anatomic structures,[2] and that familiarity with fMR imaging reports enables radiologists to provide valuable information in conventional MR imaging reports. Identifying the precise locations of lesions and understanding their relation to major functional areas and the involvement of the eloquent cortex contribute to good surgical planning and positive postoperative outcomes.[3] Basic skill in functional brain imaging may particularly improve the quality of work performed by radiologists involved in cancer care. Conventional brain scans of oncologic patients frequently show edema and postoperative changes that may lead to distortion of expected brain anatomy.[4–6] In addition, it is important to remember that the presence of pathologic conditions such as seizures or tumors can affect the functional organization of the brain (see separate article, elsewhere in this issue).[7–10]

PRIMARY SENSORIMOTOR CORTEX
Specific Anatomic Structures

The primary motor and sensory cortices occupy the pericentral region of the brain, which consists of 2 parallel gyri: the precentral gyrus (preCG) and postcentral gyrus (postCG), which are separated by the central sulcus (CS) (Fig. 1). The CS extends superiorly toward the medial interhemispheric surface of the brain and inferiorly

Funding information: National Institutes of Health (NIH): NIH-NIBIB R01 EB022720 (Makse and Holodny, principal investigators [PIs]), NIH-NCI R21 CA220144 (Holodny and Peck, PIs), NIH-NCI U54 CA137788 (Ahles, PI), NIH-NCI P30 CA008748 (Thompson, PI).

[a] Department of Radiology, Memorial Sloan Kettering Cancer Center, 1275 York Avenue, New York, NY 10065, USA; [b] Instituto do Câncer do Estado de São Paulo (ICESP), Rua Vergueiro, 5400, ap 232 torre 01 Vila Firminiano Pinto, São Paulo-SP 04272-000, Brazil

* Corresponding author. Rua Vergueiro, 5400, ap 232 torre 01 Vila Firminiano Pinto, São Paulo-SP 04272-000, Brazil.

E-mail address: raquel.moreno@hc.fm.usp.br

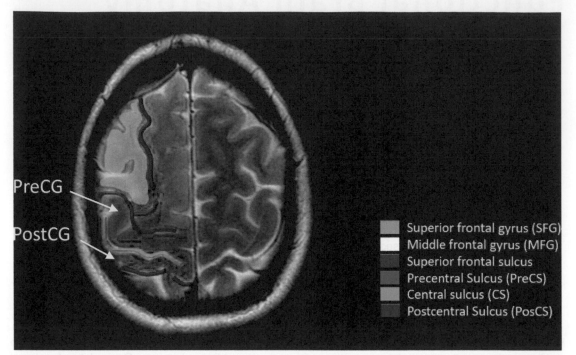

Fig. 1. Anatomic landmarks for localization of the primary sensorimotor cortex, located at the precentral gyrus and postcentral gyrus.

toward the Sylvian fissure. At the upper end of the CS, the preCG and postCG fuse together to form the paracentral lobe. At the lower end of the CS, the preCG and postCG also fuse together to form the subcentral gyrus, which is located just above the Sylvian fissure.[11]

Fig. 1 presents anatomic landmarks of the frontal and parietal lobes that facilitate the localization of the preCG and postCG on conventional MR imaging images[1,11]:

1. Superior frontal gyrus (SFG): Horizontally oriented, roughly rectangular, forms the uppermost margin of the frontal lobe.
2. Middle frontal gyrus (MFG): Horizontally oriented, undulant shape, usually merges with the anterior face of the preCG.
3. Superior frontal sulcus (SFS): Separates the SFG from the MFG; at its posterior end, the SFS bifurcates to form the superior precentral sulcus.
4. Precentral sulcus (PreCS): Anterior margin of the preCG.
5. Postcentral sulcus (PosCS): Posterior margin of the posCG.

It is important to bear in mind that these sulci are frequently discontinuous and imagining the path they generally follow may help radiologists to identify important regional structures.

Anatomic Organization

The sensory and motor systems are both organized topographically at the precentral and postcentral gyrus, respectively. This organization means that each portion of the body has a specific location on the cortex,[12,13] which is represented in a topographically organized map known as the "homunculus." Because the amount of cortex represented in the homunculus is proportional to the degree of precision or discrimination necessary for optimal function of its representative body part, the resultant maps are distorted to emphasize the face, lips, fingers, and hands.

The classic version of the motor and sensory homunculus places the foot and leg in the superior aspect of the preCG directly adjacent to the interhemispheric fissure with a small region for the trunk lateral to the legs, followed by regions representing the fingers and hands. The most inferior and lateral segments represent the lips and face.[1,12] The hand motor area is another important anatomic reference for localization of the primary motor cortex, and is located at the most posterior aspect of an area with an upside-down omega shape in the preCG known as the "reverse omega" (Ω) (**Fig. 2**). Combining localization of the hand motor area with previous knowledge of the specific parts of the motor homunculus helps radiologists

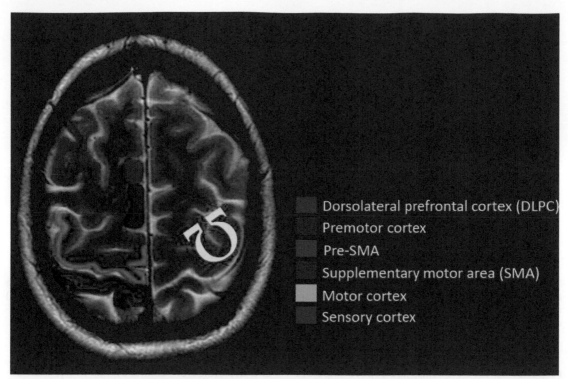

Dorsolateral prefrontal cortex (DLPC)
Premotor cortex
Pre-SMA
Supplementary motor area (SMA)
Motor cortex
Sensory cortex

Fig. 2. Axial T2-weighted image of the sensorimotor cortex with functional areas labeled in the right hemisphere. The "reverse omega" in the left hemisphere marks the specific location of the hand motor function at the posterior cortex of the central region of the precentral gyrus (PCG).

to predict which motor function may be compromised when a lesion is present in the preCG and to choose which fMR imaging paradigm should be performed on each patient.[14]

In cases in which anatomy is significantly distorted due to edema, mass effect, or postoperative changes, accurate identification of the "reverse omega" may be extremely difficult (**Fig. 3**). In such cases, visualization of functional activation in the presumed hand motor area plays a key role in defining which motor tasks may be compromised and should be presurgically evaluated. It is also important to understand that the "functional" part of the preCG (the part that is actually involved in generating movement) is located on the posterior bank of the preCG. This true both physiologically and in fMR imaging (**Fig. 4**).

PRIMARY MOTOR CORTEX

The primary motor cortex initiates voluntary movement through the corticospinal tract, which also receives contributions from the premotor cortex, supplementary cortex, and somatosensory cortex. A large percentage of corticospinal tract fibers cross in the pyramidal decussation and connect

to motor neurons in the contralateral spinal cord to trigger movement.[6] The motor cortex also connects to the cerebellum and brain stem. Through this network, subcortical regions and other cortical areas influence the input and output of the primary motor cortex. A lesion in the primary motor cortex generally results in contralateral motor weakness.[1]

PRIMARY SOMATOSENSORY CORTEX

The central processing of tactile and nociceptive stimuli takes place in the primary somatosensory cortex.[15] Fine-touch and proprioception inputs reach these cortical areas through the dorsal column–medial lemniscus pathway, and information regarding pain, temperature, and touch reach these cortical areas through the lateral and ventral spinothalamic tracts.[1,6] Early areas of activation after tactile and nociceptive stimuli are located in the postcentral gyrus (**Fig. 5**). The primary somatosensory cortex simultaneously receives information from other cortical regions and subcortical areas that modify the output response from this region, similar to the operation of the primary motor cortex.[1,15]

Although a complex and hierarchical organization within the somatosensory cortices occurs in

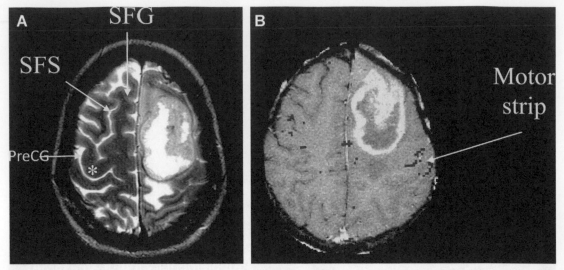

Fig. 3. Patient with an expansile tumor in the left lobe distorting local anatomy. The anatomic landmarks are easily identifiable on the right side on the axial conventional MR imaging T2 sequence (*A*): reverse omega (*) in the right PCG, SFG, SFS. By contrast, on the left side, the tumor seems to invade the expected motor area. However, fMR imaging (*B*) reveals that the motor strip in the left PCG is actually displaced backwards.

response to tactile stimuli, nociceptive impulses activate a single area in the somatosensory cortex and are immediately redirected to the primary cortex and to temporal lobe limbic structures. This difference in the organization of both modalities may reflect that pain perception requires reactions to

and avoidance of harmful stimuli rather than sophisticated sensory capacities.[15]

FOOT MOTOR AREA

The localization of the foot motor homunculus in the presurgical setting is of extreme clinical

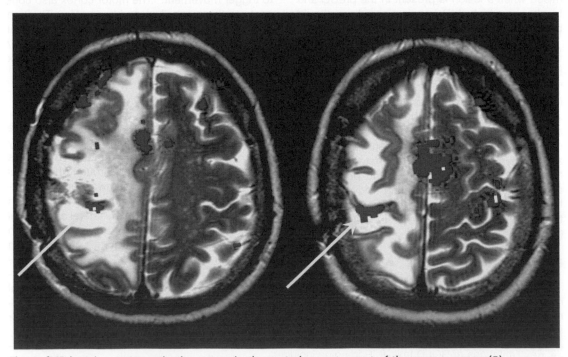

Fig. 4. fMR imaging motor activation occurs in the posterior-most aspect of the reverse omega (Ω).

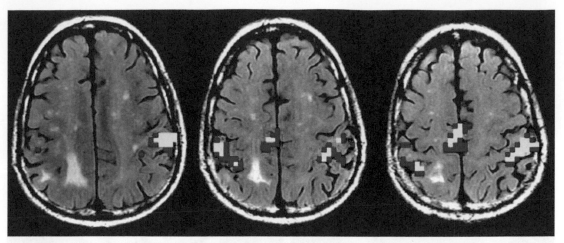

Fig. 5. Example of activation of the primary somatosensory cortex during left hand passive sensory task. The sensory fMR imaging demonstrated that the area of fluid-attenuated inversion recovery hyperintensity in the right parietal lobe did not involve the right somatosensory cortex of the hand.

importance, especially in patients with brain tumors in the frontoparietal region. Iatrogenic damage to the foot motor area and resultant paresis of the leg can render a patient wheelchair-bound or bed-bound. These conditions may be more debilitating than paresis of the nondominant hand or arm, which are commonly mapped by fMR imaging for surgical planning. By contrast, corticobulbar fibers from the contralateral hemisphere often compensate for iatrogenic compromise of the face and tongue homunculus.

The foot motor homunculus is located at the high frontoparietal convexity of the brain in the most medial aspect of the preCG and directly adjacent to the interhemispheric fissure. As this

area is usually tucked under the superior sagittal sinus, it is quite difficult to approach intraoperatively and to confirm the exact area of foot motor activation by direct cortical stimulation. Therefore, fMR imaging plays a key role in correctly identifying the foot motor area in the preoperative setting (Fig. 6).

Accurate delimitation of the foot motor area on conventional MR imaging is limited due to a lack of a discernible anatomic landmarks. The CS, which may help guide readers, often does not reach the hemispheric fissure. Furthermore, there is no sulcus between the foot motor homunculus and the supplementary motor area (SMA), which makes the distinction of the foot

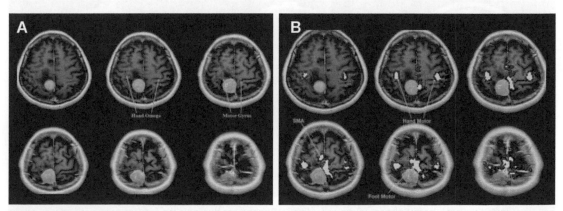

Fig. 6. Axial T1-weighted without (A) and with (B) co-registered functional MR images obtained during a bilateral finger-tapping and foot motor paradigm. fMR imaging places the extra-axial lesion just posterior to the primary motor cortex, including the foot motor portion of the motor homunculus. Edema extends to involve both the precentral and superior frontal gyri.

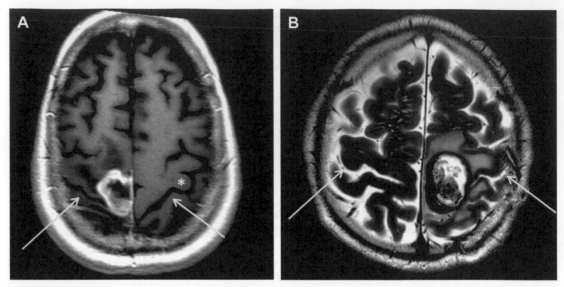

Fig. 7. Brain tumors located in the foot motor area. The "reverse omega" (*) and the CS (*arrows*) are usually located in the posterior half of the brain scans, as in (*A*). With anterior inclination of the head, as in (*B*), the same structures are displaced anteriorly. Different head positions often lead readers to misjudge the correct foot motor region.

motor area from the SMA even more difficult on routine MRI.

Another great difficulty in determining the location of the foot motor area is related to its high position in the brain, close to the convexity. Small displacements of the patient's head during image acquisition often result in significant differences in the position of regional anatomic references that guide readers, such as the "reverse omega" (**Fig. 7**). Finally, in patients with cancer, the

presence of edema imposes an additional challenge. Even if an expansile lesion is not located in the foot motor area, the surrounding edema in the white matter can compromise foot motor function (**Fig. 8**).

Fisicaro and colleagues[2] demonstrated that precise localization of the foot motor area is difficult even among experienced readers. In a study of neuroradiologist and nonradiologist readers, they found that identification of the foot motor

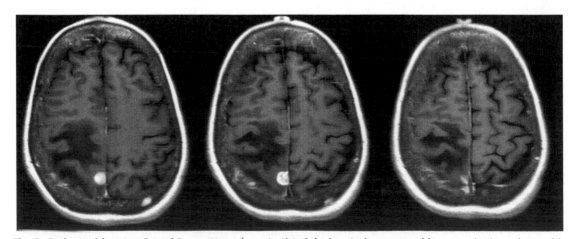

Fig. 8. Patient with extensive white matter edema in the right hemisphere caused by a meningioma located in the posterior aspect of the right parietal lobe. In this case, the compromise of the foot motor area was related to the edema rather than direct invasion.

homunculus on conventional MR imaging of patients with brain tumors was correct only 77% of the time. None of the readers, including highly experienced neuroradiologists, were correct 100% of the time, which suggests the utility of preoperative fMR imaging. In addition, readers with prior fMR imaging experience and neuroradiologists fared significantly better than readers without such expertise.

FACIAL MOTOR AREA (TONGUE AND LIPS)

The classic version of the motor homunculus places the facial motor area at the most lateral level of the preCG, in a region known as the inferior ventral precentral gyrus.[12,16] Tongue and lip movements are frequently involved in facial motions such as spoken language, mastication, and swallowing, which may be compromised in patients with injuries or lesions in the frontotemporal junction.[17]

Preoperative tongue motor-mapping with fMR imaging is of particular interest in patients with speech apraxia and difficulty finding words. In these cases, identification of the tongue motor area is important to guide intraoperative awake language mapping, in which surgeons stimulate the motor cortex to establish a current threshold and map language localization. The primary aim of the fMR imaging in such cases is in fact language-related.[12]

The bilateral angular gyrus, supramarginal gyrus, and parts of the operculum in the frontal and temporal lobes have been demonstrated to be common areas of activation for facial and tongue movements.[17] Other brain areas are also involved in facial movement within a complex facial motor network, such as the primary motor cortex (M1), the SMA, the insula, and the cerebellum. These areas seem to be highly activated during facial motor tasks and to modulate facial motor output.[17]

SUPPLEMENTARY MOTOR AREA

Not all patients with lesions in the perirolandic cortex are referred for motor strip localization. Many patients with medial frontal lesions undergo preoperative fMR imaging to localize the SMA. This area is located in the posterior aspect of the SFG; however, its anatomic boundaries are vague, making preoperative localization with fMR imaging essential. Even with fMR imaging, accurate identification and lateralization of the activated SMA can be challenging, as its midline position, its lack of specific anatomic structure, and the smoothing

of fMR imaging data impose additional difficulties in mapping this area.

The SMA has traditionally been divided into 2 major areas: the SMA proper (motor SMA) and the pre-SMA (language SMA), which is located just anterior to the SMA (Fig. 9). However, it is important to bear in mind that their functions are nuanced, their borders are indistinct and functionally variable, and they likely represent a continuum rather than discrete anatomic areas.[1,18]

The SMA proper is responsible for planning motor movements, and the pre-SMA is responsible for linguistic planning, which is further discussed in the "language" section of this article. Evidence indicates that the SMA also plays a role in other functions, such as sensation, speech expression, listening comprehension, posture, and working memory.[19]

General Anatomic Borders

The anatomic boundaries of the dorsomedial functional regions are poorly defined. The SMA occupies the dorsomedial aspect of the SFG, which is located immediately anterior to the foot motor representation. The SMA is bounded medially by the interhemispheric falx, laterally by the premotor cortex, and inferiorly by the cingulate sulcus and cingulate gyrus. The lateral and posterior borders of the SMA consist of the PreCS, which separates the SMA from the leg area in the primary motor cortex.[20] There are no sharp borders between the medial posterior aspect of the SMA and the foot motor region. The anterior margin of the SMA is also less demarcated and is defined by a

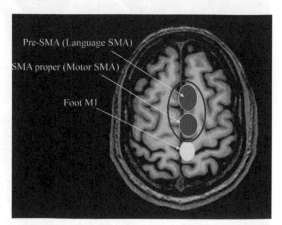

Fig. 9. The SMA. The SMA is subdivided into 2 portions: the more anterior area has a linguistic role (pre-SMA or language SMA), and the more posterior area subserves motor planning (SMA proper or the motor SMA). The expected location of the foot motor area is also indicated.

perpendicular line through the corpus callosum rostrum. A vertical line through the posterior aspect of the anterior commissure roughly differentiates the rostral from the caudal SMA.

Anatomic Organization

The relationships between distinct functional subregions within the SMA and the topographic distribution of these subregions have been intensely investigated. Recent studies have suggested a somatotopic organization in which, from anterior to posterior, the SMA represents the head, trunk, upper extremity, and lower extremity.[1]

Using various fMR imaging motor, sensory, and language tasks, Chung and colleagues[19] demonstrated the tendency of the anterior and rostral aspects of the ipsilateral SMA to activate during word generation and working memory tasks. By contrast, the contralateral SMA tended to activate during motor and heat sensory tasks, particularly in its caudal and posterior portions.[19]

SUPPLEMENTARY MOTOR AREA PROPER

The SMA proper receives inputs from the motor, premotor, and sensory cortices and provides a wide array of outputs, including outputs to the primary motor cortex, basal ganglia, thalamus, subthalamic nucleus, brain stem, contralateral SMA, and cervical motor neurons (primarily contralaterally). Projections from the SMA join those from the premotor cortex and compose approximately one-third of the corticospinal tract.[1] The SMA proper is involved in planning, coordination, laterality, and initiation of movement, particularly of complex hand motions and action sequences that involve both sides of the body.

The SMA is usually the first area to be activated in motor tasks performed in fMR imaging studies. Bilateral finger-tapping primarily results in precentral and SMA activations, whereas toe tapping primarily activates the medial aspects of the motor gyrus (**Fig. 10**).[12,21]

Unilateral resection of the SMA may result in "SMA syndrome," which is characterized by contralateral global akinesia with normoflexia or hyporeflexia and a normal tonus with preservation of extremity muscle strength. Mutism is also associated with SMA syndrome. A notable feature of SMA syndrome is that the symptoms are temporary and usually completely resolve within weeks or months, leaving only a disturbance in alternating bimanual movements.

Lesions of the dominant SMA such as tumors or anterior cerebral artery infarctions result in abulia, gait apraxia, and transient weakness.[1,19] SMA lesions (**Fig. 11**) can also result in "alien limb" syndrome, in which spontaneous movements of the limb, such as grasping, are uncontrollable by the patient, often countering the patient's attempted goal-directed motion.

LANGUAGE

The ability to communicate properly through language is an essential consideration for the

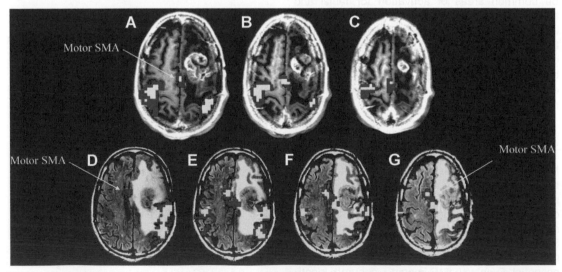

Fig. 10. Bilateral hand motor task in patient with a heterogeneous tumor in the left frontal lobe. The SMA proper (motor SMA), located in the dorsomedial aspect of the frontal lobes (*arrows*), is preserved. Analysis of both contrast-enhanced (*A–C*) and FLAIR (*D–G*) images is important in cases of high-grade glioma where the compromise of eloquent brain areas is determined by invasion of the enhanced portions of the tumor.

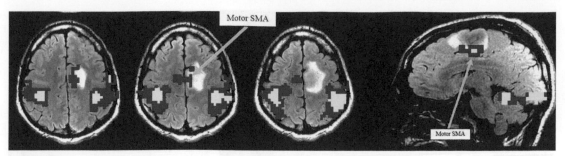

Fig. 11. In cases of low-grade tumor, the compromise of the SMA proper (motor SMA) is determined by extension of the fluid-attenuated inversion recovery hypersignal into the area of activation in the dorsomedial aspect of the left frontal lobe during bilateral hand motor task.

neurosurgeon when planning the patient's postoperative quality of life. For this reason, the potential loss of language function after neurosurgery plays a key role in the surgeon's decision whether or not perform a surgery, especially in patients with lesions in and around the language-dominant hemisphere, and in epilepsy surgeries.[11,22]

In the past, mapping functional language areas relied on invasive procedures such as the Wada test (intracarotid amytal injection), or intraoperative direct cortical stimulation. An additional, relatively new technique that can also be used to identify language function preoperatively is transcranial magnetic stimulation.[11,23,24] Functional MR imaging, a noninvasive and repeatable method, has been increasingly used to determine the areas of the cortex involved in functioning of speech.[22,25] Preoperative fMR imaging findings have come to play a key role in the neurosurgeon's decision to perform a biopsy, a subtotal resection, or a maximal resection using awake craniotomy.[26]

Current clinical fMR imaging of language relies primarily on hemispheric language dominance and spatial localization of language areas, as well as their relationship to adjacent brain tumors.[12,22] Because most of the population is right-handed, language areas reside in the left hemisphere in most individuals. More recent studies have explored language dominance in populations with different demographic characteristics including handedness, age, gender, multilingualism, and the presence of diseases.[27] Detailed clinical information before the performance of fMR imaging contributes to a more accurate interpretation of its results.

Specific Anatomic Structures

Classic functional neuroanatomy locates the motor output of language in the left inferior frontal gyrus (Broca area) (**Fig. 12**) and the perception of language in the posterior temporal lobe (Wernicke

area) (**Fig. 13**).[11] However, recent fMR imaging and neuroscientific studies have demonstrated that additional areas are commonly activated during language tasks, including the dorsolateral prefrontal cortex (MFG), pre-SMA, angular and supramarginal gyri, and occasionally the additional gyri of the frontal and temporal lobes.[18,28,29]

In addition, the precise anatomic areas that subserve speech function are not well-defined, especially in the case of the Wernicke area. Furthermore, there is considerable variability among individuals in the anatomic specialization of language anatomy. As a result, we discuss these areas in terms of frontal and temporal systems.[12]

Productive Speech: Frontal Language Areas (Broca Area)

The frontal speech language areas are centered on the inferior frontal gyrus (IFG) of the left hemisphere (Brodmann areas 44 and 45). The IFG has an overall triangular configuration, hence its synonym, "triangular gyrus." The inferior frontal sulcus (IFS) courses above the IFG, bifurcates into the inferior preCS, and thereby separates the triangular IFG from the MFG above and the preCG behind. The anterior horizontal and anterior ascending rami of the Sylvian fissure extend upward into the triangular IFG, partially subdividing it into 3 portions: the pars orbitalis, which abuts the orbital gyri of the frontal lobe; the pars triangularis in the center; and the pars opercularis, which forms the anteriormost portion of the frontal operculum. Together, the 3 parts of the IFG resemble an oblique letter "M."[11] Language is primarily located in the pars triangularis and the pars opercularis.

Lesions in this area produce an expressive aphasia often called "Broca aphasia." Most commonly, patients with Broca aphasia perform well on measures of speech comprehension but

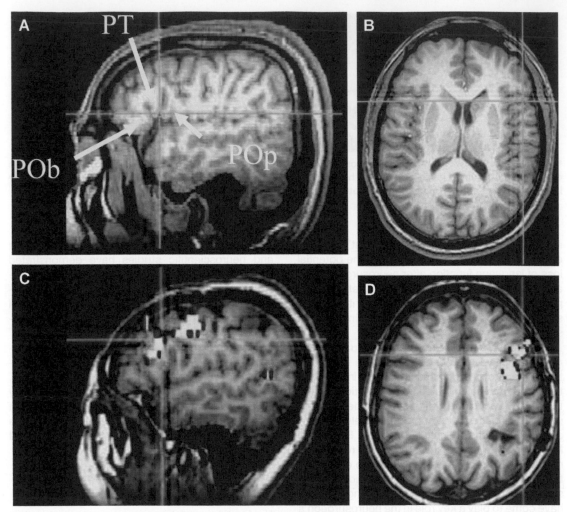

Fig. 12. Broca area on conventional and functional brain MR imaging scans. Sagittal (*A*) is the best plane to visualize the subdivisions of the IFG. POb, pars orbitalis; PT, pars triangularis; Pop, pars opercularis. The coordinates point to the expected location of the Broca area on the axial conventional image (*B*). Language tasks performed during fMR imaging (*C, D*) better determine the specific individual activated areas.

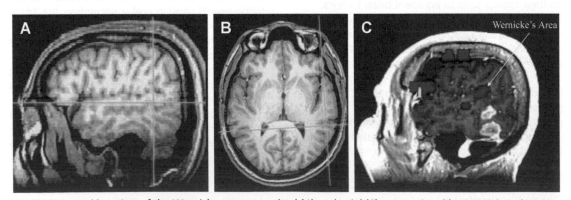

Fig. 13. Expected location of the Wernicke area on sagittal (*A*) and axial (*B*) conventional brain MR imaging. Usually the activation is seen at the posterior STG, better visualized in (*A*). However, this is one of the most variable areas of activation among individuals. (*C*) fMR imaging demonstrates the localization of the Wernicke area and its relationship to the tumor.

display agrammatic or telegraphic speech such as simplified, staccatolike sentences.[12] In addition to grammatical disorder, Broca aphasia often involves a motor deficit (language apraxia) with reduced verbal fluency, disturbances in speech speed, and melody and articulation errors.[30]

Receptive Speech: Temporal Language Areas (Wernicke Area)

The dominant temporal speech areas are primarily located in the posterior superior temporal gyrus of the left hemisphere (Brodmann area 22). However, activation in this area is variable, and frequently appears at the angular gyrus and other posterior superior temporal areas.

The superior temporal gyrus (STG), along with the middle and inferior temporal gyri, comprise most of the temporal lobe and outline the inferior and lower lateral convexities of the brain. The STG is limited superiorly by the Sylvian fissure and inferiorly by the superior temporal sulcus (STS). The STG and the middle temporal gyrus extend posteriorly and then swing upward to join with the parietal lobe. The STS courses parallel to the posterior horizontal and the posterior ascending rami of the Sylvian fissure, hence its synonym, the "parallel sulcus." The posterior portion of the STS is directed superiorly and is sometimes called the "angular sulcus."[11]

Lesions in this area produce fluent aphasias in which the patient speaks with normal inflection, rate, and cadence, but with impaired meaning (Fig. 14). In order of least complexity, fluent aphasias may be caused by alterations in auditory

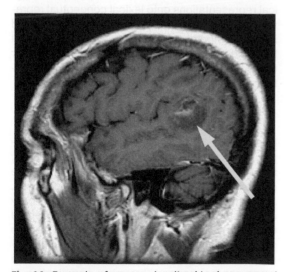

Fig. 14. Example of a tumor localized in the expected Wernicke area of activation: the posterior-most aspect of the STG.

phonological recognition (auditory verbal agnosia), verbal memory, or the capacity for lexical-semantic association. Lesions in this area may also result in word-finding difficulty and impaired confrontation naming (picture naming). Fluent aphasias often involve a degree of anosognosia, that is, the patient seems unaware of the deficit.[12,30]

LANGUAGE LATERALITY INDEX

As mentioned previously, significant evidence has demonstrated that language is predominantly mediated by the left cerebral hemisphere in the majority of the population, a phenomenon known as hemispheric specialization.[31] There is some debate about how complete this specialization is, particularly in left-handed people, in whom fMR imaging maps of language are more likely to display codominance (bi-hemispheric) or right hemisphere dominance.[12]

As determination of hemispheric brain dominance for language is essential to establishing surgical candidacy and planning, an objective measurement was developed to facilitate such classification called the language laterality index (LLI). This metric also plays a key role in the treatment of patients with slow-growing and relapsing tumors in whom translocation of speech to the nondiseased hemisphere has been reported.

The LLI is a ratio measure based on the difference between the number of active fMR imaging voxels in language functional areas from each hemisphere divided by the total activity across the hemispheres according to the following formula:

$$LLI = \left(\frac{L - R}{L + R}\right)$$

where L = vol of activation of the left Broca area and R = vol of activation of the right Broca area. The final classification is given as follows (Fig. 15):

1. LLI greater than 0.2: Left-dominant
2. 0.2 < LI < −0.2: Codominant
3. LI < −0.2: Right-dominant

Several methodological factors should be taken into account when interpreting LLI values or comparing values between subjects,[27] including the paradigms performed and the functional map statistical analysis.[22,26,32] Although the exact types of paradigms and statistical thresholds used vary from one institution to the next, in general multiple tasks, both receptive and expressive speech paradigms and a spectrum of P values should be used to ensure reliability and accuracy.

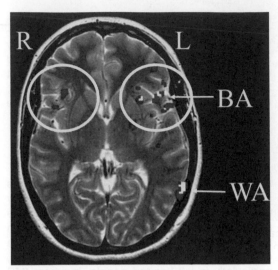

Fig. 15. The LLI is an objective measurement of the difference in activation between the left and right Broca areas. LLI = (L−R)/(L + R), where L = volume of activation of the left Broca area and R = vol of activation of the right Broca area.

A single task or threshold may produce false negative results.[12,22] Quantification of the contribution of the left and right hemispheres, localization of volumes of interest within each hemisphere, thresholding LLI values, choice of activation, baseline conditions, and reproducibility of LLI values are other factors that must be taken into account.[27]

Normal Organization of Language: Dorsal and Ventral Streams of Language

Recent studies indicate that receptive and expressive language centers and their connections are much more complex than the classic descriptions of Paul Broca (1861) and Wernicke-Geschwind (1965).[30] The integration between multiple interconnected cortico-subcortical language networks has been intensely investigated in recent decades, especially after the development of functional neuroimaging in the 1980s.[28] The most widely accepted model, recently proposed by Hickok and Poeppel,[33] is a dual-stream model of speech processing similar to previous descriptions of the organization of visual function and other sensory systems. In this model, a ventral stream processes speech signals for comprehension and a dorsal stream maps sensory or phonological representations to articulatory networks of the frontal lobe. Hickok and Peoppel[33] also propose a strong left-lateralization of the dorsal stream and assume that the ventral stream is largely bilaterally organized.

The earliest stage of cortical speech processing occurs bilaterally in the peri-Sylvian region, but not necessarily symmetrically. This stage involves spectrotemporal analysis, which is carried out bilaterally in auditory cortices in the supratemporal plane, as well as bilateral phonological-level processing and representation that involves the middle to posterior portions of the STS.[33] At this level, the acoustic speech signal and other sensory modalities transform into a conceptual representation through several processing steps that will not be discussed here.[34] Subsequently, the system diverges into 2 broad systems: the dorsal pathway that maps the sensory or phonological representations onto articulatory motor representations (phonological system), and the ventral stream that maps the same information onto lexical conceptual representations (the lexical-semantic system). The conceptual network is widely distributed.[33]

In the dorsal pathway, the signal travels from an area around the Sylvian fissure at the parietotemporal boundary (sensorimotor interface) through the supramarginal gyrus to the articulatory network in the frontal lobe, including the inferior premotor cortex, the posterior IFG, and the insula. The major fiber tract of the dorsal stream is the superior longitudinal fasciculus/arcuate fasciculus. The receptive language area in the parietotemporal junction probably includes the classic posterior temporal (Wernicke area), and the more anterior locations in the frontal lobe probably involve the well-known expressive language area (Broca area).[1,33]

The ventral stream mediates higher-level comprehension and maps sensory or phonological representations onto lexical conceptual representations. This pathway connects the middle and inferior temporal gyri with the anterior temporal lobe and ventrolateral prefrontal cortex. The major tracts of the ventral stream are the inferior occipitofrontal fasciculus and the extreme capsule.[35]

SECONDARY LANGUAGE AREAS

Besides the aforementioned major language centers and their network of complex connections, there are many secondary areas that activate consistently during language fMR imaging tasks. Although most of these areas are classically described as "nonessential," it is well accepted that their contribution to speech function can be significant, and their role in linguistics is increasingly well-defined. These other language-critical areas can be mapped through a combination of different language tasks performed during preoperative fMR imaging.[29] Their accurate localization is important, as their preservation contributes to a higher quality of life after surgery.[12]

In the section that follows, we list the major secondary language areas and briefly describe their anatomic localization and their main functional contribution to the language process. For further discussion, please refer to the bibliographic references.

Pre-Supplementary Motor Area (Supplementary Speech Area or Language Supplementary Motor Area)

Location
The pre-SMA is located anterior to the SMA within the dorsal aspect of the SFG (Brodmann cortical area 6) (Fig. 16). Studies indicate that language-related functions are predominantly located on the left side; however, the extent to which language activates the pre-SMA is variable and is not yet well-established.[1,19,36]

Function
Activation of the pre-SMA has been demonstrated during word generation and working memory tasks, especially when initiating and sequencing motor movements for speech.[37] There is also evidence that the SMA is involved in the modulation and expression of speech, speech initiation, the maintenance of speech fluency and volume, and listening comprehension. Resection of the nondominant SMA can also inhibit speech, and in cases of unilateral SMA damage, the resulting aphasia usually recovers postoperatively over weeks or months. These functions indicate the bilateral contribution of the SMA in the generation of speech. Aphasia caused by left middle cerebral artery infarction may prompt compensation by reorganization of speech function to the left SMA.[19]

Posterior Middle Frontal Gyrus (Exner Area)

Location
The Exner area is located at the posterior extent of the MFG, just anterior to the frontal eye fields. This region compounds the dorsolateral prefrontal cortex (Fig. 17) and is fundamental in cognitive processes such as working memory and executive skill, which are also recruited during use of language.[37]

Function
The Exner area is involved in transforming phonological representations of words into the motor commands for producing their written forms.[37] Studies have demonstrated the involvement of the Exner area primarily in handwriting, and also in reading and naming. Reversible alexia and agraphia have been reported after selective resection of the posterior MFG.

Angular Gyrus

Location
The angular gyrus is a horseshoe-shaped gyrus that caps the most distal portion of the STS, where the STS swings upward into the posterior portion of the inferior parietal lobule. Along with the supramarginal gyrus, the angular gyrus comprises most of the inferior parietal lobule.

Function
The angular gyrus is involved in reading and other complex language skills related to transitioning between written and spoken forms of language, including interpretation. Studies have also reported involvement of the angular gyrus in semantic processing and handwriting, as damage to this area seems to cause unintelligible writing or repetition of words.[37]

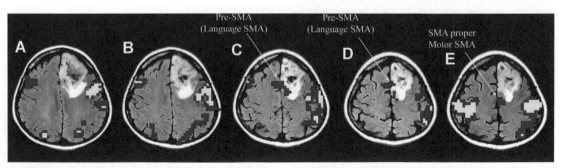

Fig. 16. Low-grade tumor compromising pre-SMA (language SMA). Semantic fluency tasks (*A–D*) demonstrate that the area of fluid-attenuated inversion recovery hypersignal invades the most anterior aspect of the SMA (*arrow*). The posterior aspect of the SMA proper (motor SMA) was preserved, as evidenced in the bilateral hand motor task (*E*).

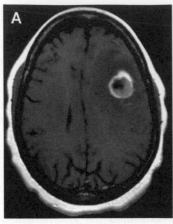
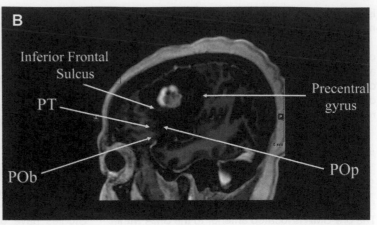

Fig. 17. Brain tumor located in the left MFG, a secondary language area. It can be difficult to precisely localize the lesion on the axial plane (*A*). The sagittal plane (*B*) facilitates visualization of anatomic landmarks: pars orbitalis (POb), pars triangularis (PT), pars opercularis (POp), IFS, and PCG. Lesion is located immediately above the Broca area. Functional MR imaging is essential in cases located in the MFG (middle frontal gyrus) to determine if there is invasion of primary language areas.

Basal Temporal Language Area

Location
The basal temporal language area is a region in the basal temporal lobe, particularly the fusiform, inferotemporal, and parahippocampal gyri.

Function
This area is involved in associating meaning with words, and is probably also related to a range of other language tasks such as visual and auditory naming, auditory comprehension, reading, repetition, and spontaneous speech, as demonstrated by interruption of this function during cortical stimulation.

Auditory Cortex and Heschl Gyrus

Location
The auditory functional areas are roughly located in the superficial posterior and superior surface of the temporal lobe. The primary auditory cortex is centered in the mid-aspect of the superior temporal plane, most precisely in the transverse temporal gyri (Heschl gyrus) (**Fig. 18**). The secondary auditory cortex has been demonstrated to be localized in the surrounding areas, in the posterior two-thirds of the superior temporal lobe and in the cortex extending medially into the posterosuperior aspect of the Sylvian fissure. The major areas related to this function are the anterior and posterior temporal planum.[1]

Function
The primary auditory cortex activates bilaterally and symmetrically with auditory presentation during language tasks, especially during auditory responsive naming.[12,38] Damage to projections from the secondary auditory cortex into the posterior Sylvian fissure results in pure word deafness with preserved nonspeech hearing.[1] The frontal/motor system is not central to speech recognition, although it may modulate auditory perception of speech.[34]

Right Hemisphere Language Areas

Processing the emotional content of language (prosodic information) associated with speech has been demonstrated to rely primarily on right-hemispheric mechanisms. The contribution of the right Broca homolog to left hemisphere language areas includes prosody, discourse, and processing of syntax. With the right ventral premotor cortex, the right Broca area has been suggested to promote recovery of speech in nonfluent aphasia since 1877.[39] The right hemisphere also has important language function in metaphors and puns, multilayered meaning, and music and singing.

VISUAL SYSTEM

Vision is the ability to infer complex 3-dimensional attributes of objects from an analysis of relatively simple visual afferences such as luminance, spectral contrast, orientation, movement, and binocular disparity. Visuospatial attention is a complex, active, dynamic process in which particular details of the visual scene are selected and passed into our consciousness and memory.[11,12] Because vision is the most essential of our senses, its importance and complexity are often most appreciated when compromised due to damage or illness.[40] Focal pathologies and treatment-

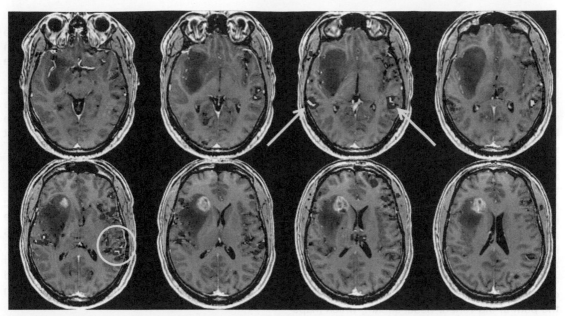

Fig. 18. Language task performed during a preoperative fMR imaging in a patient with a tumor in the right frontal lobe and extensive edema in the ipsilateral hemisphere. The superior images reveal early bilateral activation of the Heschl's gyrus with auditory presentation (*yellow arrows*). The inferior images demonstrate simultaneous activation of the left Wernicke area (*yellow circle*).

induced damage to the visual system can produce a wide spectrum of vision deficits that affect patients' routines and quality of life. The severity and location of the damage in the visual field, along with the patient's lifestyle and occupation, determine how much vision loss the individual can tolerate.

From a clinical perspective, fMR imaging study of visual areas provides retinotopic maps of the visual cortex that predict potentially iatrogenic deficits from invasive surgical and radiation treatment of nearby brain tumors, arteriovenous malformations, or epileptic foci.[40,41] These maps are particularly important for lesions located at the occipital and parietal lobes, as these lesions may involve the optic radiations. A combination of fMR imaging and diffusion tensor imaging displaying visual cortical areas and optic radiations would minimize postoperative injuries. Performance of visual tasks in fMR imaging exams also plays a role as an internal control of the fMR imaging study; if other task paradigms fail, fMR imaging vision mapping under passive viewing conditions can successfully reveal fMR imaging activation.[40]

Specific Anatomic Structures

Vision is a highly complex task involving multiple systems that are subcomponents of an overall network of areas and pathways. Recent neuroimaging studies have demonstrated that there are multiple functional visual areas in the brain. These areas constitute up to one-third of the cerebral cortex and are not limited to the calcarine fissure of the occipital lobe, as previously believed. In fact, vision-related areas extend throughout the entire occipital lobe, into adjacent portions of the parietal and temporal lobes, and even into remote locations in the frontal lobes.[11,12,40]

Visual cortex

Visual information is transferred from the retina to the lateral geniculate nucleus and subsequently to the visual cortex following a well-known retinotopic organization. This organization is determined by the spatial arrangements of points in the visual field (which are upside-down and backward due to the optical properties of the cornea and lens) and by the organization of the photoreceptor cells in the eyes. This retinotopic organization is preserved at subsequent stages of neural processing within the visual system, which produces a neuroanatomical map of the visual field at each level.[12]

Visual information from the inferior portions of the visual field reaches the primary visual cortex primarily through the optic radiations. The cortex representation of this area is located above the calcarine sulcus. Information from the superior portions of the visual field reaches the inferior portion of the primary visual cortex under the calcarine sulcus primarily through the Meyer's loop in the temporal lobe. Posteriorly, the optic radiations merge with the inferior lateral fasciculus and inferior fronto-occipital fasciculus to form a compact bundle near the ventricular trigone.[12]

The primary visual area (V1, Brodmann area 17) is located in the striate cortex, which is located around the calcarine fissure. However, the precise site of the striate cortex is variable. The calcarine sulcus runs obliquely in an anterosuperior direction from the occipital pole to its junction with the parieto-occipital sulcus to form the anterior calcarine sulcus. The calcarine sulcus generally presents a variation of different configurations and positions, and often appears disrupted and asymmetrical.[11] Virtually all types of visual information are initially processed in V1 (the primary visual area) and in V2 (the second visual area), to which it is intimately connected. The lingual gyrus and fusiform gyrus, which are located on the ventral aspect of the occipital lobe, make up the ventral occipitotemporal cortex (VOTC). The VOTC forms the path of the ventral visual stream, which maps perceptions of the visual system to conceptual representations.[1]

Central visual field (fovea) and peripheral visual field

The visual field consists of a binocular portion that is viewed simultaneously by both eyes and supports stereoscopic vision and 2 monocular portions at the lateral periphery of the field that are seen by each individual eye.[12] The center of the gaze (fovea) is represented at or near the posterior tip of the occipital lobe. Most peripheral fields are represented anteriorly near the junction of the calcarine and parieto-occipital sulci, extending in depth through the cerebrum, and the deepest activations on the lower bank of the calcarine fissure are next to the tectum.[12,42] However, there is a major distortion in this map insofar as small portions of the field increasingly close to the center of gaze are represented in larger cortical areas of V1, which reflects the critical importance of foveal vision. Neurons in V1 have the smallest receptive fields of all visual areas.

Normal Organization of Vision: Dorsal and Ventral Streams

The dual-stream model of vision was first conceptualized by Ungerleider,[43] who hypothesized that dual and distinct computational streams proceeded in parallel, with the dorsal stream analyzing spatial position and the ventral stream identifying objects.

The initial understanding of those streams was of 2 anatomically distinct, serial, hierarchical pathways that begin in the striate cortex (area V1) and that follow successively higher stages of visual processing. However, recent studies have demonstrated that these pathways are more likely to be recurrent, highly interactive, and connected "in parallel." Different areas within a hierarchical stage represent alternate concurrent processing pathways with a faster dorsal pathway and a slower ventral stream. Each major stream has multiple functional substreams, and the 2 streams have many cross-connections so that they can interact frequently.[12,44]

Dorsal stream ("Where" pathway)

The dorsal stream is classically described as connecting the striate cortex V1 area to the parietal lobe (V5), and runs primarily through V3A and the middle temporal visual complex (hMT+). This pathway is associated with motion, representation of object locations, and control of the eyes and arms, especially when visual information is used to guide saccades or reaching. The dorsal stream is involved in vision for action.

Ventral stream ("What" pathway)

The initial understanding of the ventral stream was of a pathway connecting the occipital lobe to the anterior part of the inferior temporal cortex (area IT) in which complex object representations are formed. Studies have demonstrated that this stream also has connections with the medial temporal lobe, limbic system, and dorsal stream. The ventral stream is associated with object and face recognition and form representation. The connection between the ventral stream with the limbic system has been associated with visual memory, mediating the formation of visual memories, and emotional attachments to images.[1]

Extrastriate Visual Areas

Most visual areas are grouped into the 2 major streams, each of which is responsible for identifying a particular type of stimulus and containing a retinotopic map of the visual field (though with decreasing precision at later stages of processing). The function of these streams within the complex visual network is presented below.

Dorsal stream

1. V3: Global motion, coherent motion, weaker connections with V1, stronger connections with inferior temporal lobe.
2. hMT+ (also known as V5/middle temporal lobe-MT): Complex of subareas located laterally near the temporoparieto-occipital junction at about the same dorsoventral level as the calcarine sulcus medially. Involved in perception of motion and guidance of eye movements.

Receives inputs from V1, V2, V4, lateral geniculate nucleus, and pulvinar.

Ventral stream

1. V4/VO: Ill-defined in humans. Roughly located in the posterior fusiform gyrus or anterior lingual gyrus. Associated with color and form processing.
2. Fusiform face area (FFA): Located in the right fusiform gyrus. Related to identification of particular faces. Injury to the FFA can result in prosopagnosia, the inability to recognize familiar faces with the retained ability to identify that a visual stimulus is a face.[1]
3. Visual word form area: Located in the left fusiform gyrus. Injuries in this area cause pure alexia in which a patient cannot read but can speak and comprehend language normally.[1]

From a clinical neuroimaging perspective, functional mapping of individual components of these systems has not been routine, in part because such functional losses are well tolerated by most individuals, and because selective activation of these components requires additional fMR imaging paradigms that can be time-consuming. However, advances in techniques for more detailed functional mapping improves clinical knowledge of the complexity of visual areas beyond V1/V2.

Function
The clinical significance of the "cortical magnification" of central visual field areas is that large lesions in the posterior visual cortex can cause relatively small field defects, and patients infrequently complain about these losses. In clinical practice, such small deficits can be hard to demonstrate on confrontational neurologic testing but can significantly impair visual functions such as reading that require high-acuity vision. During fMR imaging studies, clinically optimized stimuli, behavioral tasks, analysis, and displays permit identification of cortical subregions supporting high-acuity central vision that is critical for reading and other essential visual functions.[40]

Beyond the medial occipital cortex (V1/V2), cortical lesions may result in the loss of some vision-related functions while sparing others, depending on which areas and anatomic interconnections are affected. Examples include prosopagnosia, cerebral achromatopsia, alexia, and akinetopsia. We must bear in mind, however, that selective deficits are not caused by damage to a specific visual area.[12] Such deficits result from insults to the sub-unities of an extended network, as in the lesions described below:

1. Lesions of components of the dorsal stream can cause optic ataxia or visually guided misreaching. Specifically, lesions in hMT+ can cause a rare inability to perceive movement, a failure of ocular pursuit, and inaccurate saccades to moving targets.[12]
2. Bilateral lesions involving the VOTC can result in agnosia of other types of visual objects with the retained ability to identify the objects using other sensory inputs.
3. Injuries to the lingual gyri and portions of the fusiform gyri can result in loss of color vision (cerebral achromatopsia) and the inability to name colors (color anomia) while sparing visual acuity.

DISCLOSURE

R.A. Moreno has nothing to disclose. A.I. Holodny is the Owner/President of fMR imaging Consultants, LLC, a purely educational entity.

REFERENCES

1. Hill VB, Cankurtaran CZ, Liu BP, et al. A practical review of functional MRI anatomy of the language and motor systems. AJNR Am J Neuroradiol 2019;40(7): 1084–90.
2. Fisicaro RA, Jiao RX, Stathopoulos C, et al. Challenges in identifying the foot motor region in patients with brain tumor on routine MRI: advantages of fMRI. AJNR Am J Neuroradiol 2015;36(8):1488–93.
3. Gupta A, Shah A, Young RJ, et al. Imaging of brain tumors: functional magnetic resonance imaging and diffusion tensor imaging. Neuroimaging Clin N Am 2010;20(3):379–400.
4. Holodny AI, Nusbaum AO, Festa S, et al. Correlation between the degree of contrast enhancement and the volume of peritumoral edema in meningiomas and malignant gliomas. Neuroradiology 1999; 41(11):820–5.
5. Lin X, Lee M, Buck O, et al. Diagnostic accuracy of T1-weighted dynamic contrast-enhanced-MRI and DWI-ADC for differentiation of glioblastoma and primary CNS lymphoma. AJNR Am J Neuroradiol 2017; 38(3):485–91.
6. Pan C, Peck KK, Young RJ, et al. Somatotopic organization of motor pathways in the internal capsule: a probabilistic diffusion tractography study. AJNR Am J Neuroradiol 2012;33(7):1274–80.
7. Holodny AI, Schulder M, Ybasco A, et al. Translocation of Broca's area to the contralateral hemisphere as the result of the growth of a left inferior frontal glioma. J Comput Assist Tomogr 2002; 26(6):941–3.
8. Petrovich NM, Holodny AI, Brennan CW, et al. Isolated translocation of Wernicke's area to the right hemisphere in a 62-year-man with a temporo-

parietal glioma. AJNR Am J Neuroradiol 2004;25(1): 130–3.

9. Fisicaro RA, Jost E, Shaw K, et al. Cortical plasticity in the setting of brain tumors. Top Magn Reson Imaging 2016;25(1):25–30.

10. Li Q, Dong JW, Del Ferraro G, et al. Functional translocation of Broca's area in a low-grade left frontal glioma: graph theory reveals the novel, adaptive network connectivity. Front Neurol 2019; 10:702.

11. Stippich C. Clinical functional MRI: presurgical functional neuroimaging. Springer; 2015.

12. Holodny AI. Functional neuroimaging: a clinical approach. CRC Press; 2008.

13. Overduin SA, Servos P. Distributed digit somatotopy in primary somatosensory cortex. Neuroimage 2004; 23(2):462–72.

14. Mallela AN, Peck KK, Petrovich-Brennan NM, et al. Altered resting-state functional connectivity in the hand motor network in glioma patients. Brain Connect 2016;6(8):587–95.

15. Ploner M, Schmitz F, Freund H-J, et al. Differential organization of touch and pain in human primary somatosensory cortex. J Neurophysiol 2000;83(3): 1770–6.

16. Klingner CM, Volk GF, Brodoehl S, et al. Time course of cortical plasticity after facial nerve palsy: a single-case study. Neurorehabil Neural Repair 2012;26(2): 197–203.

17. Xiao F-L, Gao P-Y, Qian T-Y, et al. Cortical representation of facial and tongue movements: a task functional magnetic resonance imaging study. Clin Physiol Funct Imaging 2017;37(3):341–5.

18. Peck KK, Bradbury M, Psaty EL, et al. Joint activation of the supplementary motor area and presupplementary motor area during simultaneous motor and language functional MRI. Neuroreport 2009; 20(5):487–91.

19. Chung GH, Han YM, Jeong SH, et al. Functional heterogeneity of the supplementary motor area. AJNR Am J Neuroradiol 2005;26(7):1819–23.

20. Potgieser ARE, de Jong BM, Wagemakers M, et al. Insights from the supplementary motor area syndrome in balancing movement initiation and inhibition. Front Hum Neurosci 2014;8:960.

21. Peck KK, Bradbury MS, Hou BL, et al. The role of the supplementary motor area (SMA) in the execution of primary motor activities in brain tumor patients: functional MRI detection of time-resolved differences in the hemodynamic response. Med Sci Monit 2009; 15(4):MT55–62.

22. Ruff IM, Petrovich Brennan NM, Peck KK, et al. Assessment of the language laterality index in patients with brain tumor using functional MR imaging: effects of thresholding, task selection, and prior surgery. AJNR Am J Neuroradiol 2008;29(3): 528–35.

23. Krieg SM, Sollmann N, Hauck T, et al. Functional language shift to the right hemisphere in patients with language-eloquent brain tumors. PLoS One 2013; 8(9):e75403.

24. Brennan NP, Peck KK, Holodny A. Language mapping using fMRI and direct cortical stimulation for brain tumor surgery: the good, the bad, and the questionable. Top Magn Reson Imaging 2016; 25(1):1–10.

25. Peck KK, Bradbury M, Petrovich N, et al. Presurgical evaluation of language using functional magnetic resonance imaging in brain tumor patients with previous surgery. Neurosurgery 2009;64(4):644–52. discussion 52–3.

26. Chen CM, Hou BL, Holodny AI. Effect of age and tumor grade on BOLD functional MR imaging in preoperative assessment of patients with glioma. Radiology 2008;248(3):971–8.

27. Seghier ML. Laterality index in functional MRI: methodological issues. Magn Reson Imaging 2008;26(5): 594–601.

28. Del Ferraro G, Moreno A, Min B, et al. Finding influential nodes for integration in brain networks using optimal percolation theory. Nat Commun 2018;9(1): 2274.

29. Li QG, Del Ferraro G, Pasquini L, et al. Core language brain network for fMRI language task used in clinical applications. Netw Neurosci 2020;4(1): 134–54.

30. Jiménez de la Peña MM, Gómez Vicente L, García Cobos R, et al. Neuroradiologic correlation with aphasias. Cortico-subcortical map of language. Radiologia 2018;60(3):250–61.

31. Bradshaw AR, Bishop DV, Woodhead ZV. Methodological considerations in assessment of language lateralisation with fMRI: a systematic review. PeerJ 2017;5:e3557.

32. Chang CY, Peck KK, Brennan NM, et al. Functional MRI in the presurgical evaluation of patients with brain tumors: characterization of the statistical threshold. Stereotact Funct Neurosurg 2010;88(1): 35–41.

33. Hickok G, Poeppel D. The cortical organization of speech processing. Nat Rev Neurosci 2007;8(5): 393–402.

34. Hickok G. The functional neuroanatomy of language. Phys Life Rev 2009;6(3):121–43.

35. Saur D, Kreher BW, Schnell S, et al. Ventral and dorsal pathways for language. Proc Natl Acad Sci U S A 2008;105(46):18035–40.

36. Lou W, Peck KK, Brennan N, et al. Left-lateralization of resting state functional connectivity between the presupplementary motor area and primary language areas. Neuroreport 2017;28(10):545–50.

37. Benjamin CF, Walshaw PD, Hale K, et al. Presurgical language fMRI: mapping of six critical regions. Hum Brain Mapp 2017;38(8).4239 55

38. Kwon JS, McCarley RW, Hirayasu Y, et al. Left planum temporale volume reduction in schizophrenia. Arch Gen Psychiatry 1999;56(2):142–8.

39. Gupta SS. fMRI for mapping language networks in neurosurgical cases. Indian J Radiol Imaging 2014;24(1):37–43.

40. DeYoe EA, Raut RV. Visual mapping using blood oxygen level dependent functional magnetic resonance imaging. Neuroimaging Clin N Am 2014;24(4):573–84.

41. Gabriel M, Brennan NP, Peck KK, et al. Blood oxygen level dependent functional magnetic resonance imaging for presurgical planning. Neuroimaging Clin N Am 2014;24(4):557–71.

42. Stenbacka L, Vanni S. fMRI of peripheral visual field representation. Clin Neurophysiol 2007;118(6):1303–14.

43. Ungerleider LG. Two cortical visual systems. Anal Vis Behav 1982;549–86.

44. Goelman G, Dan R, Keadan T. Characterizing directed functional pathways in the visual system by multivariate nonlinear coherence of fMRI data. Sci Rep 2018;8(1):16362.

The Problem of Neurovascular Uncoupling

Shruti Agarwal, PhD[a], Haris I. Sair, MD[a,b], Jay J. Pillai, MD[a,c],*

KEYWORDS

- Motor activation • Neurovascular uncoupling • Presurgical mapping

KEY POINTS

- Brain tumor-induced neurovascular uncoupling (NVU) may adversely affect the reliability of both task and resting state BOLD functional MRI.
- Cerebrovascular reactivity (CVR) mapping using breath hold techniques is an effective method for assessing NVU potential.
- Various resting state fMRI metrics are being investigated as potential alternatives to CVR mapping for assessment of NVU risk.
- Novel methods for mitigation of NVU are being investigated including the resting state fMRI metric amplitude of low frequency fluctuations (ALFF).

INTRODUCTION

In 1991, Belliveau and colleagues[1] demonstrated that cerebral activation could be imaged using high-resolution MR imaging. Before this study, low-resolution PET studies had documented that regional cerebral blood flow increased near areas of neuronal activity in the human brain. This study obtained echo-planar images of the primary visual cortex before and after administration of a gadolinium bolus and calculated cerebral blood volumes in the stimulated versus nonstimulated states; the subtracted functional maps showed increased activity. The method used by Belliveau and colleagues[1] is now called dynamic susceptibility contrast (DSC) MR imaging. In 1992, Ogawa and colleagues[2] described blood oxygen level dependent (BOLD) imaging, which forms the basis for current functional MR imaging (fMR imaging). BOLD contrast was first demonstrated in a rodent model in 1990 and was first used for fMR imaging

activation studies of the human visual cortex in 1992. Instead of using gadolinium contrast, BOLD exploited different magnetic properties of oxygenated and deoxygenated blood to detect changes in regional blood flow. Regional arteriolar dilatation with increased capillary filling occurs in response to brain activation, and therefore more oxygenated blood is supplied than is required for the brain's immediate metabolic needs. In other words, the degree of regional cerebral blood flow (CBF) increase is significantly greater than the degree of concurrent increase in the cerebral metabolic rate of oxygen consumption ($CMRO_2$) during neuronal activity compared with the baseline. A decrease in the relative concentration of deoxyhemoglobin in active cortex reduces the T2/T2* shortening effects of deoxyhemoglobin with a resultant net increase in the BOLD signal in activated areas. In 1995, Biswal and colleagues[3] demonstrated correlations among groups of brain

[a] Division of Neuroradiology, The Russell H. Morgan Department of Radiology and Radiological Science, Johns Hopkins University School of Medicine, 600 North Wolfe Street, Baltimore, MD 21287, USA; [b] The Malone Center for Engineering in Healthcare, The Whiting School of Engineering, Johns Hopkins University, Baltimore, MD, USA; [c] Department of Neurosurgery, Johns Hopkins University School of Medicine, 1800 Orleans Street, Baltimore, MD 21287, USA
* Corresponding author. Division of Neuroradiology, The Russell H. Morgan Department of Radiology and Radiological Science, The Johns Hopkins Hospital, Phipps B-100, 600 North Wolfe Street, Baltimore, MD 21287.
E-mail address: jpillai1@jhmi.edu

Neuroimag Clin N Am 31 (2021) 53–67
https://doi.org/10.1016/j.nic.2020.09.003

regions that were known to function together even at rest (in the absence of the task performance). These findings suggested that networks of brain regions that activate or deactivate together during tasks maintain connectivity signatures that can be detected and studied even at rest. In 2001, Raichle and Snyder[4] discovered that brain energy consumption is increased by less than 5% of its baseline energy consumption while performing a focused mental task.

Reliance on BOLD signal to represent activity in the brain has certain limitations.[5] One major limitation is that the BOLD signal is an indirect measurement of neuronal activity. In the presence of brain tumors or other focal brain lesions, the coupling between neuronal activity and the hemodynamic changes occurring in the adjacent vasculature is often disrupted, which is called neurovascular uncoupling (NVU).[6,7] NVU is a major challenge when interpreting BOLD fMR imaging activation maps in the focal brain lesion setting, as it may lead to decreased or even absent activation in the electrically active, essential, functional (ie, eloquent) cortex.[8–11]

This article reviews the challenges of brain tumor–induced NVU, which is a critical limitation of BOLD fMR imaging. NVU affects both task-based and resting state fMR imaging analysis in cases of structural brain lesions.[12,13] We focus our discussion on MR imaging approaches to detecting NVU and mitigating its effects.

THE PROBLEM OF NEUROVASCULAR UNCOUPLING IN CLINICAL FUNCTIONAL MR IMAGING

Due to its feasibility and robustness, task-based BOLD fMR imaging has been established as the standard of care for noninvasive presurgical planning for patients with brain tumors and other focal brain lesions.[14–22] In fMR imaging, the brain is repeatedly imaged while the subject is at rest and then while the subject performs an active sensory, motor, or cognitive task to localize activated brain functional regions related to the task. The resulting difference between the signals acquired during the rest period and the active period represents activation within the network of interest, which is useful in presurgical planning. Near brain tumors, the normally tight coupling between neuronal activity and the hemodynamic changes occurring in the adjacent vasculature may become disrupted due to abnormalities in the tumor vasculature or in the vessels near the tumor. This, in turn, results in abnormally decreased or absent task-related fMR imaging activation in the cortical regions near tumors,

despite the patient's ability to adequately perform tasks that would normally activate the network of interest involving these cortical regions (**Figs. 1–3** for an example of how NVU affects the language system and **Figs. 4** and **5** for an example of how NVU affects the motor system).[23–27] This abnormally decreased activation is called false negative activation. This differs from loss of expected activation in a similar cortex associated with a functional network in eloquent cortical destruction by tumor, where the patient's ability to perform an fMR imaging task would be impaired in conjunction with the loss of activated BOLD signal. In the latter scenario, the absence of detectable BOLD signal would be considered a true negative rather than the result of NVU. Additionally, it is essential to differentiate unexpected lack of activation due to NVU from true cortical reorganization (neural plasticity). Clinically meaningful reorganization of language areas has been described multiple times in the neurosurgical literature.[23–27] Ulmer and colleagues[11] coined the term "pseudo-reorganization" to describe the effect of NVU on fMR imaging in brain tumors to distinguish this phenomenon form "true" reorganization. Thus, when present, NVU disguises, and may therefore result in the unintentional surgical resection of, the eloquent cortex. This could result in permanent postsurgical neurologic disability related to injury of cortical regions in the affected inadequately activated network.[9]

NVU is a critical limitation of clinical fMR imaging and has been widely studied in task-based fMR imaging.[9–11,28–32] NVU may be present in variable degrees, which results in variable degrees of reduction of expected ipsilesional BOLD activation in eloquent cortical regions, including complete absence of detectable activation in severe cases. NVU may result from disruption of any component of the normal neurovascular coupling cascade (NCC), which is composed of a series of biochemical steps at the cellular level, including (proximally) neurotransmitters released from activated neurons to astrocytes and (distally) chemical mediators that directly act on vascular smooth muscle of arterioles that are responsible for regulating blood flow.[7,33] Preclinical studies have suggested that tumors may induce remodeling of the extracellular matrix, changes in endothelial cells, and changes in endothelial-associated astrocytes that disrupt the NCC.[34–37] Studies have suggested that the disruption of NCC in the vicinity of high-grade gliomas is primarily caused by tumor angiogenesis that results in compromise of normal cerebral autoregulatory capacity in the tumoral and peritumoral regions.[29,30] However, in cases of infiltrating low-grade gliomas, disruption of the NCC

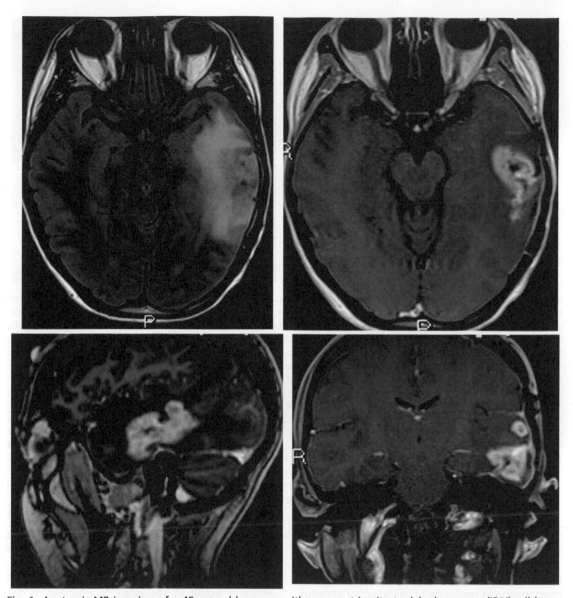

Fig. 1. Anatomic MR imaging of a 45-year old woman with recurrent isocitrate dehydrogenase (IDH) wild-type (IDH R132H mutant protein absent), O^6-Methylguanine-DNA-methyltransferase (MGMT)-unmethylated World Health Organization Grade IV glioblastoma involving the left temporal lobe. The top row displays T2 fluid-attnuated inversion recovery axial images on the left and postcontrast T1-weighted image on the right. The bottom row displays postcontrast sagittal (*left*) and coronal (*right*) images. These images display thick irregular nodular peripheral enhancement and central necrosis; histopathology revealed active tumor.

may be caused by a different etiology such as glio-vascular uncoupling between astrocytic contacts and surrounding microvasculature.[38–40] While the mechanisms underlying brain tumor–induced NVU are not yet completely understood, potential for NVU can be detected via demonstration of regionally impaired cerebrovascular reactivity (CVR),[41] which is an indication of microvascular hemodynamic dysfunction.

DETECTION OF BRAIN TUMOR–INDUCED NEUROVASCULAR UNCOUPLING USING CEREBROVASCULAR REACTIVITY MAPPING

CVR is the response of cerebral blood vessels to a physiologic challenge. CVR is quantified as the change in CBF per change in vasoactive stimulus. Near tumors, the vasoactivity of cerebral vessels decreases, resulting in reduced capacity for dynamic blood flow control in response to increasing

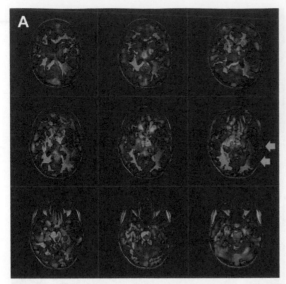
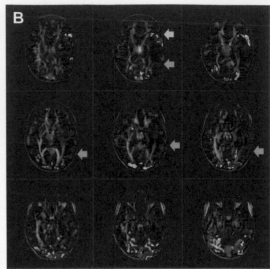

Fig. 2. (*A*) displays a BH CVR map overlaid on noncontrast T1-weighted 3-dimensional magnetization prepared rapid acquisition gradient echo (MPRAGE) anatomic images (thresholded at 0.5 BOLD % signal change, color-coded in blue) for the 45-year old woman with glioblastoma described in Fig. 1. Notice the areas of abnormally reduced regional CVR in the left temporal lobe along the lateral cortical margins of the hypointense infiltrative tumor, as shown by green arrows, compared with the normal contralateral intact right temporal cortical CVR. This indicates NVU. (*B*) presents an overlaid multicolor-coded language activation map displaying activation from 7 different language tasks (silent word generation in *red*, sentence completion in *yellow*, noun-verb semantic association task in *magenta*, rhyming in *light blue*, sentence listening comprehension in *orange*, passive story listening in *purple*, and object naming in *green*, differentially thresholded). In addition, color fractional anisotropy maps from diffusion tensor imaging are overlaid using standard Red, Green, Blue (RGB) convention; these display infiltration of temporal lobe white matter tracts, including the green inferior fronto-occipital and inferior longitudinal fasciculi as well as the uncinate fasciculus. Notice that there is robust Broca's area activation (*light blue arrow*) in the left inferior frontal gyrus, but in the expected areas of Wernicke's area and other temporal lobe receptive language activation (*green arrows*) where reduced regional CVR is noted, absolutely no activation is seen on any task. This is direct evidence of NVU in the language network, as the patient was able to perform all 7 tasks without any difficulty that would suggest receptive aphasia.

neural demand. Thus, regional reduction in CVR serves as a biomarker for potential NVU.

CVR mapping can be performed using BOLD fMR imaging, which measures changes in blood oxygenation in response to vasodilatory stimulus. Davis and colleagues[42] described the BOLD signal change in terms of CBF and $CMRO_2$. Under the most CVR challenges (ie, hypercapnic conditions), changes in $CMRO_2$ relative to the baseline are negligible, leading to effectively linear dependence of BOLD on CBF, making BOLD suitable for CVR measurement. Previously, the vasodilating drug acetazolamide was used for CVR assessment[43]; however, for clinical assessment of CVR, noninvasive methods are preferred.

Hypercapnia (increased blood carbon dioxide [CO_2] concentration) has been widely used as a noninvasive method to elicit increased blood flow via vasodilation of cerebral arteries by endothelial smooth muscle cell relaxation.[44–49] Hypercapnia can be induced via inhalation of CO_2-enriched air or breath-holding.[21,41,50,51] In the former, CO_2-enriched air is supplied through a breathing-mask to the subject during the fMR imaging scan.

CVR is calculated as the change in BOLD fMR imaging signal in response to changes in the end-tidal (ie, end expiratory) partial pressures of carbon dioxide ($etCO_2$) between the baseline and a vascular challenge condition expressed as $\Delta\%$ BOLD/$\Delta etCO_2$. The measurement of $etCO_2$ is an important component for accurately assessing CVR.[52] Complex and expensive computerized systems have been developed to implement increased $etCO_2$ stimuli[53,54] via dynamic end-tidal forcing[55,56] and prospective targeting.[57,58] In addition, simple respiratory circuits that administer fixed concentrations of inspired gases have been developed.[59–61] Although issues have been raised regarding the performance of simple circuits using fixed inspired concentrations,[62,63] this method is less expensive and easier to use. A recent review article by Fisher[52] offers a detailed comparison between the fixed inspired concentration methods

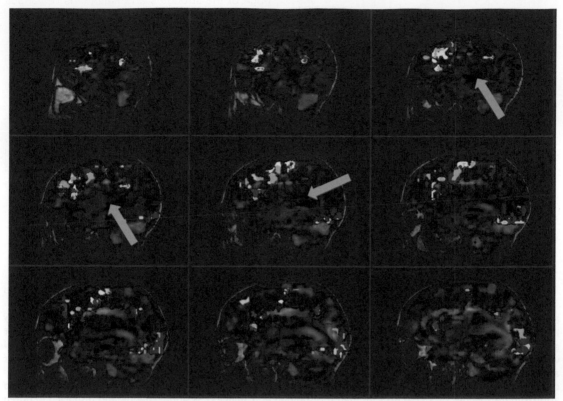

Fig. 3. This figure displays language activation maps and BH CVR map for the patient described in **Figs. 1** and **2**, but displays sagittal rather than axial noncontrast T1-weighted anatomic overlays. The green arrows point to the regions of abnormally decreased CVR where Wernicke's area activation would be expected but is absent due to tumor-related NVU.

and computer-controlled prospective targeting methods regarding issues such as complexity/simplicity, effectiveness, and cost. A detailed technical review of CVR MR imaging mapping with CO_2 challenges is provided in a recent article by Liu and colleagues.[64]

Regardless of the type of system used, CO_2 inhalation methods require MR imaging-compatible equipment that may not be available with all scanners. Not all patients can tolerate the breathing-mask, and these patients are often excluded from CO_2 breathing studies for CVR measurements. Thus, breath-holding (BH) BOLD fMR imaging is becoming a popular alternative for CVR mapping.[19,21,41–43,65–75] BH CVR mapping has been demonstrated to be comparable in CVR assessment to gas inhalation techniques[71] and is thus considered reliable.[66] Several clinical studies have been performed using BH to assess vascular health.[19,21,28,41,67,68,76–78] In these studies, BH CVR is measured by inducing hypercapnia using a block design paradigm under physiologic monitoring.[73] Paced breathing between BH blocks provides a consistent baseline condition from which

the BH signal response can be more accurately extracted.[79]

Pillai and Zaca[68] have demonstrated the advantages of BH CVR mapping over T2* DSC MR gadolinium perfusion imaging in the detection of NVU in brain tumors of varying grades. T2* DSC MR perfusion imaging has been widely used to assess tumor vascularity.[80] Hemodynamic variables such as elevated relative cerebral blood volume and relative CBF are associated with tumor neovascularity in high-grade gliomas,[29,81] which are indirectly associated with impaired CVR due to NVU. However, in low-grade gliomas, in which regional hyperperfusion is not generally seen, static perfusion imaging is not a reliable option to assess NVU.[68] Therefore, BH CVR mapping may be an effective tool to evaluate both high-grade and low-grade gliomas.[28,67,68,82,83] In another study by Iranmahboob and colleagues,[76] BH maps based on peak-to-trough were used to characterize vascular reactivity in brain tumors (ie, BOLD signal between the minimal signal seen at the end of a deep inhalation at the beginning of a BH block and maximal signal seen at the end of

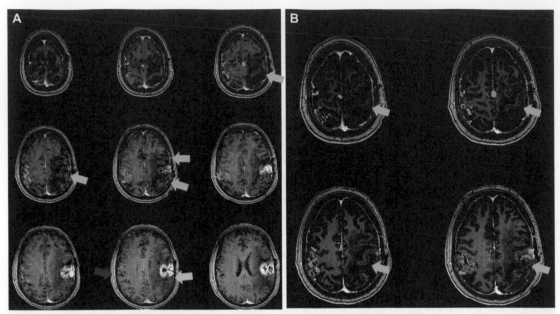

Fig. 4. This figure (and **Fig. 5**) display images of a patient with left perirolandic World Health Organization Grade IV glioblastoma (58-year-old man with profound right facial weakness and expressive aphasia but only mild right arm weakness). (*A*) presents a composite motor task fMR imaging activation map overlaid on postcontrast T1-weighted 3D MPRAGE images. Hand opening/closing and bilateral simultaneous sequential finger tapping tasks are color-coded as blue and magenta, respectively, and a vertical tongue movement face motor task is color-coded as green. All task activation maps were thresholded at 0.35 clustered cross-correlation (equivalent to approximate T-values of 3.7). A BH CVR map thresholded at 0.50 BOLD % signal change and displayed in green is superimposed on the composite motor activation map. Notice the extensive area of abnormally reduced CVR in the left frontal and parietal lobes (*yellow arrows*), including in the left precentral and postcentral gyri, where activation is expected in the hand motor (*yellow arrows*) and face motor (*light blue arrow*) areas. No activation is seen in these areas despite the patient's ability to perform the hand motor tasks, albeit with mild weakness, and this reflects tumor-induced NVU. The absent face motor activation on the vertical tongue movement task reflects true negative activation rather than false negative activation due to NVU, as the tumor presumably destroyed the face motor cortex and the patient presented with dense facial paralysis. Notice the normal contralateral right face motor activation (*red arrow*). (*B*) shows only the composite motor activation map without CVR overlay. The yellow arrows depict the areas of absent but expected hand motor activation, indicative of NVU.

a BH block). The study evaluated 16 patients with various grades of gliomas and demonstrated that vascular reactivity maps in patients with brain tumor appear to be caused by a mechanism other than gadolinium enhancement. Hsu and colleagues[83] evaluated 6 low-grade gliomas and one high-grade glioma and found that BH mapping can demonstrate differential cerebrovascular response between normal tissue and cerebral glioma. Another study by Zaca and colleagues[82] compared BH CVR maps with clinical task fMR imaging activation maps of 12 patients with histologic diagnosis of Grade II glioma who performed multiple motor tasks and a BH task. Sensorimotor activation maps and BH CVR maps were compared in 2 automatically defined regions of interest involving the ipsilesional and contralesional perirolandic cortex, respectively. The study demonstrated that BH CVR maps were effective for assessment of NVU affecting the primary sensorimotor cortex in patients with low-grade perirolandic tumors. Pillai and Mikulis[41] extensively described the details of BH CVR map acquisition and analysis in the clinical setting, including applications for presurgical mapping. See **Figs. 2–4** for examples of how BH CVR maps can be useful in detecting NVU.

Despite its advantages, BH BOLD fMR imaging poses several challenges. BH responses vary between populations depending on the inhalation depth before BH,[84] requiring parallel use of respiratory bellows to monitor subject compliance during the BH task.[70] Although BH signal response depends on the subject's capacity to comply with longer BH durations (resulting in more robust BH responses),[66,85] breath-holds following inspiration (ie, end-inspiration)[79] with short BH durations of 20 seconds or less[85] can

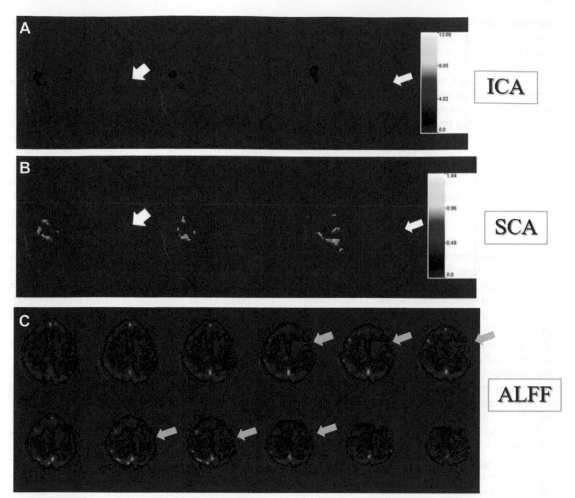

Fig. 5. This figure depicts resting state fMR imaging results for the patient described in **Fig. 4**. (*A*) (*top row*) depicts the results of independent component analysis displaying the single ICA component that best identifies the primary motor network (thresholded at z-score > 3.0). Notice the absence of synchronized BOLD signal in the affected left primary motor cortex (*white arrows*) and visualized signal in the intact right motor cortex. (*B*) (*middle row*) depicts the results of seed-based correlation (SCA) analysis using a right primary motor cortex (precentral gyral) seed region of interest (thresholded at z-score > 1.0). Again, notice the absence of expected synchronized BOLD signal fluctuations in the left primary motor cortex (*white arrows*). The bottom 2 rows (*C*) display the results of ALFF analysis (thresholded at ALFF > 0.35). Notice the abnormally decreased ALFF in the left frontal lobe, including the expected location of the left primary motor cortex (*yellow arrows*). These are 3 different manifestations of NVU-related BOLD signal loss in resting state fMR imaging. (*Adapted from* Agarwal S, Sair HI, Pillai JJ. Limitations of Resting-State Functional MR Imaging in the Setting of Focal Brain Lesions. Neuroimaging Clin N Am. 2017;27(4):645-661; with permission.)

generally be comfortably performed without reaching the subject's tolerance limit.[86] Motion artifacts tend to be increased in BH protocols.[87] BH stimulus can also vary across time points; for example, BH following inspiration is biphasic, consisting of an initial signal dip followed by a signal increase,[70,88] which is not seen in end-expiration BHs. The BH hemodynamic response is slower than neuronal task-related BOLD signal changes, as the peak occurs several seconds after the BH period; therefore, modeling the BH

response for CVR mapping is often challenging.[66,85,89–92] Birn and colleagues[92] modeled the BOLD fMR imaging signal changes resulting from BH and cued depth and rate changes with a respiration response function, which consists of an early overshoot followed by a later undershoot (peaking at approximately 16 seconds). Unfortunately, repeatability of BH fMR imaging may be limited due to variability in task performance, especially in the absence of end-tidal CO_2 measures.[66]

Resting state BOLD fMR imaging signals have been explored as a useful alternative to CVR measurements in clinical applications when CO_2-hypercapnic challenge and BH are not feasible. Kannurpatti and Biswal[93] presented the resting state fluctuation of amplitude (RSFA), a task-free marker obtained from resting state BOLD fMR imaging (rsfMR imaging) scans, as a viable CVR biomarker that may be useful in a wider population than BH techniques.[94] Various studies of BOLD amplitude changes during CO_2-hypercapnic challenge or BH indicated a strong correlation between resting state BOLD fluctuations and end-tidal CO_2 fluctuations, establishing RSFA as a strong CVR correlate.[71,94–96] Liu and colleagues[97] proposed another method for CVR mapping using rsfMR imaging that does not require gas inhalation. This approach exploits the natural variation in respiration and its influence on BOLD fMR imaging. The study demonstrated that global BOLD signal fluctuation in the frequency range of 0.02 to 0.04 Hz contains the most prominent contribution from natural variation in arterial CO_2.

RsfMR imaging has attracted wide attention as a preoperative mapping tool[98–105] due to its less stringent requirements for patient compliance.[102,104,106–110] Brain tumor-related NVU limits rsfMR imaging just as it limits clinical task-based fMR imaging.[12,13,18,98,111–117] For this reason, using rsfMR imaging as a reliable presurgical mapping tool necessitates further study of brain tumor-related NVU in rsfMR imaging.

DETECTION OF NEUROVASCULAR UNCOUPLING IN RESTING STATE FUNCTIONAL MR IMAGING

There have been considerable efforts to clinically implement rsfMR imaging in the domain of presurgical brain mapping.[98–102,118–122] Our group at Johns Hopkins has conducted various retrospective rsfMR imaging studies related to the sensorimotor network, demonstrating the prevalence of NVU affecting this network in patients with brain tumors.[12,111–113] Our recent review articles have discussed in detail methods of image acquisition, monitoring, and analysis of rsfMR imaging, as well as the impact of NVU on its application to presurgical mapping in the language network.[122,123]

Despite much exploration, there is still no consensus regarding optimal processing approaches for clinical application of rsfMR imaging.[124] In rsfMR imaging, different areas of the brain display temporally correlated BOLD signal fluctuations in the absence of task performance, and this property can be exploited to derive intrinsic brain networks known as resting state networks (RSNs).[3,125,126] The most common methods to identify RSNs are seed-based correlation analysis (SCA) and independent component analysis (ICA). In SCA, voxels within a region of interest (seed region) are selected and their average BOLD time course is correlated with that of all other voxels in the brain. Voxels showing a correlation with the seed region above a certain threshold are considered to be functionally related to the region of interest. In SCA, a priori selection of seed regions is required. In contrast, ICA is a model-free approach,[127] which separates the BOLD time courses of all voxels into different spatial components and ensures maximum statistical independence.[128] Because this is a purely data-driven approach, in contrast to the "seed region" approach, there is no clear link between components and specific brain functions. Other methods of rsfMR imaging analysis include cluster analysis and graph theoretic analysis.

Agarwal and colleagues[12] evaluated 7 patients with de novo peri-rolandic tumors who underwent comprehensive clinical fMR imaging exams for presurgical mapping with conventional 3T MR imaging. On both ICA and SCA analysis, abnormally reduced synchronized BOLD signal fluctuations were noted ipsilesionally within the primary motor network (despite intact motor function) as a manifestation of motor network NVU, as the motor network is normally a non-lateralized network.[12] Another study reported similar motor network NVU in 2 de novo brain tumor patients at ultrahigh field (7T) strength MR imaging; the higher signal-to-noise ratio was not sufficient to mitigate the effects of NVU in these patients.[13] Mallela and colleagues[116] examined functional connectivity of the primary and supplementary motor areas in 24 glioma patients using rsfMR imaging and correlated this with tumor characteristics and clinical information to characterize functional reorganization of RSNs. The study demonstrated that the decreased sensitivity of rsfMR imaging in high-grade gliomas was caused by NVU. In a recent study, Sun and colleagues[18] investigated the association between tumors, tumor characteristics, and changes in resting state connectivity using SCA in 45 glioma patients and demonstrated that differences in resting state connectivity may be caused by false negatives, possibly related to NVU. In another recent study, Lemee and colleagues[129] investigated rsfMR imaging ICA-derived RSNs versus task-based fMR imaging for language mapping with correlation with intraoperative cortical mapping during awake craniotomies in 50 adult patients. The study concluded that rsfMR imaging for presurgical language mapping allows identification of the functional brain language network with greater sensitivity than task-based fMR imaging, but with lower specificity, which may be due to NVU in the vicinity of the tumor. In another recent study, Bathla and colleagues[130] examined the resting-state functional connectivity of the supplementary motor area (SMA) in 14 brain tumor patients and compared the SMA subdivisions (pre-SMA, SMA proper, central SMA) connectivity with the motor (precentral) gyrus and language centers. All 14 patients showed connectivity between the pre-SMA and language centers and between the SMA proper and motor gyrus; 13 patients showed connectivity between the central SMA and both the language and motor areas. The only case that did not show central SMA connectivity was caused by tumor infiltration and resultant NVU.

Another way to look at resting state connectivity is through the hypothesis that intrinsic brain activity is manifested by clusters of voxels rather than single voxels. Zang and colleagues[131] proposed this hypothesis of regional homogeneity (ReHo) metrics. ReHo does not require a priori definition of regions of interest and can provide information about the local/regional activity of regions throughout the brain. Agarwal and colleagues[112] demonstrated that NVU is detectable in ReHo maps and that these findings may correlate with abnormally reduced motor fMR imaging task activation. Amplitude of low-frequency fluctuations (ALFF) and fractional ALFF (fALFF) have been used as additional rsfMR imaging analysis methods, particularly for frequency domain analysis.[132] Since rsfMR imaging focuses on spontaneous low-frequency fluctuations (<0.1 Hz) in the BOLD signal, ALFF is defined as the total power within the frequency range between 0.01 to 0.08 Hz. fALFF is defined as the ratio of the power spectrum of the low-frequency (0.01–0.08 Hz) range to that of the entire frequency range, representing the relative contribution of specific low-frequency fluctuation.[133] Our group recently demonstrated that ALFF may be sensitive enough to detect NVU in brain tumors that affect the sensorimotor network,[111] as ALFF may reflect both a lower frequency band CVR component and a higher frequency band neuronal component and may be used to mitigate the effects of NVU on task-based fMR imaging activation maps.[133] **Fig. 5** displays the effects of NVU on rsfMR imaging maps derived through ICA, SCA, and ALFF

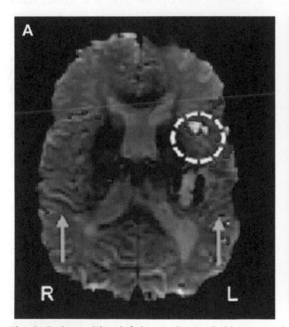
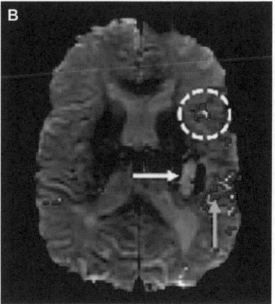

Fig. 6. Patient with a left hemispheric glioblastoma who underwent fMR imaging examination to identify the location of the primary language areas. The fMR imaging scan, which was obtained using standard methods of analysis, localized Broca's area (*white circle*) but did not localize or lateralize Wernicke's area (*green arrows*). The fMR imaging scan, which was obtained by incorporating the BH data to adjust the routine method of analysis, revealed Wernicke's area, the crucial eloquent area for optimal preoperative assessment (*green arrow*). The white arrow points to the tumor in part B.

analysis methods in a patient with left perirolandic glioblastoma.

In addition to the CVR and resting state methods, another less commonly used method to detect NVU is functional field mapping, which was first described in research applications in the human visual system.[10] This article will not describe this approach as it has not yet been applied widely to clinical NVU detection.

MITIGATION OF NEUROVASCULAR UNCOUPLING USING AMPLITUDE OF LOW-FREQUENCY FLUCTUATIONS

In a preliminary study,[112] our group enhanced the detectability of motor task activation in the ipsilesional sensorimotor cortex affected by tumor-induced NVU using ALFF from resting state fMR imaging. We observed that the average motor task activation time course in the sensorimotor cortex in contralesional (CL) and ipsilesional (IL) hemispheres of brain tumor patients were similar in periodicity; however, the relatively low amplitude of IL BOLD signal compared with CL signal reflects the effects of NVU on the IL voxels in the vicinity of the lesion. In this study, we applied an ALFF-based correction approach that utilized ratios of CL/IL ALFF values to enhance the detectability of task activation in the NVU-affected primary sensorimotor cortex.

Other approaches that have been used to mitigate the effects of NVU include a voxel-based BH CVR calibration approach and a promising recent coherence-based model that incorporates identical block design BH CVR and task-based fMR imaging activation to overcome the limitations of tumor-induced NVU.[134,135] Using this approach, Voss and colleagues[135] studied 16 patients (9 glioblastomas, one anaplastic astrocytoma, 5 low-grade astrocytomas, and 1 metastasis) and 6 healthy controls. The study used an independent measurement of NVU quantified by the BH method to adjust the BOLD fMR imaging signal in patients with brain tumors. In the patient group, adjustment of the BOLD fMR imaging scan by incorporating the BH data resulted in the identification of clinically meaningful areas of BOLD fMR imaging activation that were not seen on routine analysis (Fig. 6).

SUMMARY

This review has considered NVU-related problems affecting the reliability of presurgical mapping with task-based and resting state fMR imaging. Methods of NVU detection using CVR mapping as well as resting state fMR imaging metrics

were outlined. We also reviewed novel approaches to mitigate the effects of NVU using frequency domain resting state fMR imaging metrics. We anticipate that the challenges of presurgical brain mapping with BOLD MR imaging will be further studied and addressed by future research.

CLINICS CARE POINTS

- Neurovascular uncoupling (NVU) is a major pitfall in the interpretation of clinical functional activation maps.
- NVU is important to recognize because it can lead to spuriously decreased or even absent activation in eloquent cortex within any functional brain network.
- NVU risk can be assessed through either cerebrovascular reactivity mapping or resting state methods.

DISCLOSURE

The authors report no financial conflicts of interest.

REFERENCES

1. Belliveau JW, Kennedy DN Jr, McKinstry RC, et al. Functional mapping of the human visual cortex by magnetic resonance imaging. Science 1991; 254(5032):716–9.
2. Ogawa S, Tank DW, Menon R, et al. Intrinsic signal changes accompanying sensory stimulation: functional brain mapping with magnetic resonance imaging. Proc Natl Acad Sci U S A 1992;89(13):5951–5.
3. Biswal B, Yetkin FZ, Haughton VM, et al. Functional Connectivity in the Motor Cortex of Resting Human Brain Using Echo-Planar Mri. Magn Reson Med 1995;34(4):537–41.
4. Raichle ME, Snyder AZ. A default mode of brain function: a brief history of an evolving idea. Neuroimage 2007;37(4):1083–90 [discussion: 97–9].
5. Logothetis NK. What we can do and what we cannot do with fMRI. Nature 2008;453(7197): 869–78.
6. Villringer A, Dirnagl U. Coupling of brain activity and cerebral blood-flow - basis of functional neuroimaging. Cerebrovas Brain Met 1995;7(3):240–76.
7. Attwell D, Buchan AM, Charpak S, et al. Glial and neuronal control of brain blood flow. Nature 2010; 468(7321):232–43.
8. Holodny AI, Schulder M, Liu WC, et al. Decreased BOLD functional MR activation of the motor and sensory cortices adjacent to a glioblastoma multiforme: implications for image-guided neurosurgery. AJNR Am J Neuroradiol 1999;20(4):609–12.
9. Holodny AI, Schulder M, Liu WC, et al. The effect of brain tumors on BOLD functional MR imaging activation in the adjacent motor cortex: implications for

image-guided neurosurgery. AJNR Am J Neuroradiol 2000;21(8):1415–22.

10. DeYoe EA, Ulmer JL, Mueller WM, et al. Imaging of the functional and dysfunctional visual system. Semin Ultrasound CT MR 2015;36(3):234–48.

11. Ulmer JL, Krouwer HG, Mueller WM, et al. Pseudoreorganization of language cortical function at fMR imaging: a consequence of tumor-induced neurovascular uncoupling. Am J Neuroradiol 2003; 24(2):213–7.

12. Agarwal S, Sair HI, Yahyavi-Firouz-Abadi N, et al. Neurovascular uncoupling in resting state fMRI demonstrated in patients with primary brain gliomas. J Magn Reson Imaging 2016;43(3):620–6.

13. Agarwal S, Sair HI, Airan R, et al. Demonstration of brain tumor-induced neurovascular uncoupling in resting-state fMRI at ultrahigh field. Brain Connect 2016;6(4):267–72.

14. Peck KK, Bradbury M, Petrovich N, et al. Presurgical evaluation of language using functional magnetic resonance imaging in brain tumor patients with previous surgery. Neurosurgery 2009;64(4): 644–52.

15. Gupta A, Shah A, Young RJ, et al. Imaging of brain tumors: functional magnetic resonance imaging and diffusion tensor imaging. Neuroimaging Clin N Am 2010;20(3):379–400.

16. Gabriel M, Brennan NP, Peck KK, et al. Blood oxygen level dependent functional magnetic resonance imaging for presurgical planning. Neuroimaging Clin N Am 2014;24(4):557–71.

17. Del Ferraro G, Moreno AA-OX, Min B, et al. Finding influential nodes for integration in brain networks using optimal percolation theory. Nat Commun 2018;9:2274.

18. Sun H, Vachha B, Laino ME, et al. Decreased hand motor resting-state functional connectivity in patients with glioma: analysis of factors including neurovascular uncoupling. Radiology 2020;294(3):610–21.

19. Pillai JJ. The evolution of clinical functional imaging during the past 2 decades and its current impact on neurosurgical planning. AJNR Am J Neuroradiol 2010;31(2):219–25.

20. Petrella JR, Shah LM, Harris KM, et al. Preoperative functional MR imaging localization of language and motor areas: effect on therapeutic decision making in patients with potentially resectable brain tumors. Radiology 2006;240(3):793–802.

21. Pillai J, Zaca D, Choudhri A. Clinical impact of integrated physiologic brain tumor imaging. Technol Cancer Res Treat 2010;9(4):359–80.

22. Fox ME, King TZ. Functional connectivity in adult brain tumor patients: a systematic review. Brain Connect 2018;8(7):381–97.

23. Holodny AI, Schulder M, Ybasco A, et al. Translocation of Broca's area to the contralateral hemisphere as the result of the growth of a left inferior

frontal glioma. J Comput Assist Tomogr 2002; 26(6):941–3.

24. Petrovich NM, Holodny AI, Brennan CW, et al. Isolated translocation of Wernicke's area to the right hemisphere in a 62-year-man with a temporoparietal glioma. AJNR Am J Neuroradiol 2004; 25(1):130–3.

25. Fisicaro RA, Jost E, Shaw K, et al. Cortical plasticity in the setting of brain tumors. Top Magn Reson Imaging 2016;25(1):25–30.

26. Cho NS, Peck KK, Zhang Z, et al. Paradoxical activation in the cerebellum during language fMRI in patients with brain tumors: possible explanations based on neurovascular uncoupling and functional reorganization. Cerebellum 2018;17:286–93, 1473-4230 (Electronic).

27. Li Q, Dong JW, Del Ferraro G, et al. Functional translocation of Broca's area in a low-grade left frontal glioma: graph theory reveals the novel, adaptive network connectivity. Front Neurol 2019; 10:1664–2295.

28. Zaca D, Jovicich J, Nadar SR, et al. Cerebrovascular reactivity mapping in patients with low grade gliomas undergoing presurgical sensorimotor mapping with BOLD fMRI. J Magn Reson Imaging 2014;40(2):383–90.

29. Hou BL, Bradbury M, Peck KK, et al. Effect of brain tumor neovasculature defined by rCBV on BOLD fMRI activation volume in the primary motor cortex. Neuroimage 2006;32(2):489–97.

30. Jiang Z, Krainik A, David O, et al. Impaired fMRI activation in patients with primary brain tumors. Neuroimage 2010;52(2):538–48.

31. Fraga de Abreu VH, Peck KK, Petrovich-Brennan NM, et al. Brain tumors: the influence of tumor type and routine MR imaging characteristics at BOLD functional MR imaging in the primary motor gyrus. Radiology 2016;281:876–83, 1527-1315 (Electronic).

32. Silva MA, See AP, Essayed WI, et al. Challenges and techniques for presurgical brain mapping with functional MRI. Neuroimage Clin 2018;17: 794–803, 2213-1582 (Electronic).

33. Venkat P, Chopp M, Chen J. New insights into coupling and uncoupling of cerebral blood flow and metabolism in the brain. Croat Med J 2016; 57(3):223–38.

34. Lee J, Lund-Smith C, Borboa A, et al. Glioma-induced remodeling of the neurovascular unit. Brain Res 2009;1288:125–34, 1872-6240 (Electronic).

35. Pak RW, Hadjiabadi DH, Senarathna J, et al. Implications of neurovascular uncoupling in functional magnetic resonance imaging (fMRI) of brain tumors. J Cereb Blood Flow Metab 2017;37(11): 3475–87.

36. Montgomery MK, Kim SH, Dovas A, et al. Glioma-induced alterations in neuronal activity and

neurovascular coupling during disease progression. Cell Rep 2020;31(2):107500.

37. Hosford PS, Christie IN, Niranjan A, et al. A critical role for the ATP-sensitive potassium channel subunit K(IR)6.1 in the control of cerebral blood flow. J Cereb Blood Flow Metab 2019; 39(10):2089–95.

38. Pelligrino DA, Vetri F, Xu HL. Purinergic mechanisms in gliovascular coupling. Semin Cell Dev Biol 2011;22(2):229–36.

39. Watkins S, Robel S, Kimbrough IF, et al. Disruption of astrocyte-vascular coupling and the blood-brain barrier by invading glioma cells. Nat Commun 2014;5:4196, 2041-1723 (Electronic).

40. Chaitanya GV, Minagar A, Alexander JS. Neuronal and astrocytic interactions modulate brain endothelial properties during metabolic stresses of in vitro cerebral ischemia. Cell Commun Signal 2014;12:7, 1478-811X (Electronic).

41. Pillai JJ, Mikulis DJ. Cerebrovascular reactivity mapping: an evolving standard for clinical functional imaging. AJNR Am J Neuroradiol 2015; 36(1):7–13.

42. Davis TL, Kwong KK, Weisskoff RM, et al. Calibrated functional MRI: Mapping the dynamics of oxidative metabolism. Proc Natl Acad Sci U S A 1998;95(4):1834–9.

43. Lythgoe DJ, Williams SCR, Cullinane M, et al. Mapping of cerebrovascular reactivity using bold magnetic resonance imaging. Magn Reson Imaging 1999;17(4):495–502.

44. Fierstra J, Sobczyk O, Battisti-Charbonney A, et al. Measuring cerebrovascular reactivity: what stimulus to use? J Physiol 2013;591(23):5809–21.

45. Brian JE Jr. Carbon dioxide and the cerebral circulation. Anesthesiology 1998;88(5):1365–86.

46. Hoiland RL, Fisher JA, Ainslie PN. Regulation of the cerebral circulation by arterial carbon dioxide. Compr Physiol 2019;9(3):1101–54.

47. Vavilala MS, Lee LA, Lam AM. Cerebral blood flow and vascular physiology. Anesthesiol Clin North Am 2002;20(2):247–64, v.

48. Madden JA. The effect of carbon dioxide on cerebral arteries. Pharmacol Ther 1993;59(2):229–50.

49. Kety SS, Schmidt CF. The effects of altered arterial tensions of carbon dioxide and oxygen on cerebral blood flow and cerebral oxygen consumption of normal young men. J Clin Invest 1948;27(4): 484–92.

50. Tancredi FB, Hoge RD. Comparison of cerebral vascular reactivity measures obtained using breath-holding and CO2 inhalation. J Cereb Blood Flow Metab 2013;33(7):1066–74.

51. Blockley NP, Harkin JW, Bulte DP. Rapid cerebrovascular reactivity mapping: enabling vascular reactivity information to be routinely acquired. Neuroimage 2017;159:214–23, 1095-9572 (Electronic).

52. Fisher JA. The CO2 stimulus for cerebrovascular reactivity: fixing inspired concentrations vs. targeting end-tidal partial pressures. J Cereb Blood Flow Metab 2016;36(6):1004–11.

53. Fisher JA, Iscoe S, Duffin J. Sequential gas delivery provides precise control of alveolar gas exchange. Respir Physiol Neurobiol 2016;225:60–9, 1878-1519 (Electronic).

54. Baddeley H, Brodrick PM, Taylor NJ, et al. Gas exchange parameters in radiotherapy patients during breathing of 2%, 3.5% and 5% carbogen gas mixtures. Br J Radiol 2000;73(874):1100–4.

55. Wise RG, Pattinson KT, Bulte DP, et al. Dynamic forcing of end-tidal carbon dioxide and oxygen applied to functional magnetic resonance imaging. J Cereb Blood Flow Metab 2007;27(8):1521–32.

56. Poublanc J, Crawley AP, Sobczyk O, et al. Measuring cerebrovascular reactivity: the dynamic response to a step hypercapnic stimulus. J Cereb Blood Flow Metab 2015;35(11):1746–56.

57. Slessarev M, Han J, Mardimae A, et al. Prospective targeting and control of end-tidal CO2 and O2 concentrations. J Physiol 2007;581(Pt 3):1207–19.

58. Fisher JA, Sobczyk O, Crawley A, et al. Assessing cerebrovascular reactivity by the pattern of response to progressive hypercapnia. Hum Brain Mapp 2017;38(7):3415–27.

59. Lu H, Liu P, Yezhuvath U, et al. MRI mapping of cerebrovascular reactivity via gas inhalation challenges. J Vis Exp 2014;94:52306.

60. Tancredi FB, Lajoie I, Hoge RD. A simple breathing circuit allowing precise control of inspiratory gases for experimental respiratory manipulations. BMC Res Notes 2014;7:235, 1756-0500 (Electronic).

61. Prisman E, Slessarev M, Azami T, et al. Modified oxygen mask to induce target levels of hyperoxia and hypercarbia during radiotherapy: a more effective alternative to carbogen. Int J Radiat Biol 2007;83(7):457–62.

62. Duffin J. Measuring the respiratory chemoreflexes in humans. Respir Physiol Neurobiol 2011;177(2): 71–9.

63. Mark CI, Slessarev M, Ito S, et al. Precise control of end-tidal carbon dioxide and oxygen improves BOLD and ASL cerebrovascular reactivity measures. Magn Reson Med 2010;64(3):749–56.

64. Liu P, De Vis JB, Lu H. Cerebrovascular reactivity (CVR) MRI with CO2 challenge: A technical review. Neuroimage 2019;187:104–15, 1095-9572 (Electronic).

65. Murphy K, Harris AD, Wise RG. Robustly measuring vascular reactivity differences with breath-hold: normalising stimulus-evoked and resting state BOLD fMRI data. Neuroimage 2011; 54(1):369–79.

66. Bright MG, Murphy K. Reliable quantification of BOLD fMRI cerebrovascular reactivity despite

poor breath-hold performance. Neuroimage 2013; 83:559–68, 1095-9572 (Electronic).

67. Pillai JJ, Zaca D. Clinical utility of cerebrovascular reactivity mapping in patients with low grade gliomas. World J Clin Oncol 2011;2(12):397–403.

68. Pillai JJ, Zaca D. Comparison of BOLD cerebrovascular reactivity mapping and DSC MR perfusion imaging for prediction of neurovascular uncoupling potential in brain tumors. Technol Cancer Res Treat 2012;11(4):361–74.

69. Cohen AD, Wang Y. Improving the assessment of breath-holding induced cerebral vascular reactivity using a multiband multi-echo ASL/BOLD sequence. Sci Rep 2019;9(1):5079.

70. Thomason ME, Glover GH. Controlled inspiration depth reduces variance in breath-holding-induced BOLD signal. Neuroimage 2008;39(1): 206–14.

71. Kastrup A, Kruger G, Neumann-Haefelin T, et al. Assessment of cerebrovascular reactivity with functional magnetic resonance imaging: comparison of CO_2 and breath holding. Magn Reson Imaging 2001;19(1):13–20.

72. Blockley NP, Griffeth VE, Buxton RB. A general analysis of calibrated BOLD methodology for measuring CMRO2 responses: comparison of a new approach with existing methods. Neuroimage 2012;60(1):279–89.

73. Kastrup A, Kruger G, Glover GH, et al. Regional variability of cerebral blood oxygenation response to hypercapnia. Neuroimage 1999;10(6):675–81.

74. Ratnatunga C, Adiseshiah M. Increase in middle cerebral artery velocity on breath holding: a simplified test of cerebral perfusion reserve. Eur J Vasc Surg 1990;4(5):519–23.

75. Zhou Y, Rodgers ZB, Kuo AH. Cerebrovascular reactivity measured with arterial spin labeling and blood oxygen level dependent techniques. Magn Reson Imaging 2015;33(5):566–76.

76. Iranmahboob A, Peck KK, Brennan NP, et al. Vascular reactivity maps in patients with gliomas using breath-holding BOLD fMRI. Neuroimaging 2016;26:232–9, 1552-6569 (Electronic).

77. Peng SL, Yang HC, Chen CM, et al. Short- and long-term reproducibility of BOLD signal change induced by breath-holding at 1.5 and 3 T. Nmr Biomed 2020;33(3):e4195.

78. Muscas G, van Niftrik CHB, Sebok M, et al. Hemodynamic investigation of peritumoral impaired blood oxygenation-level dependent cerebrovascular reactivity in patients with diffuse glioma. Magn Reson Imaging 2020;70:50–6, 1873-5894 (Electronic).

79. Scouten A, Schwarzbauer C. Paced respiration with end-expiration technique offers superior BOLD signal repeatability for breath-hold studies. Neuroimage 2008;43(2):250–7.

80. Sage MR, Wilson AJ. The blood-brain barrier: an important concept in neuroimaging. AJNR Am J Neuroradiol 1994;15(4):601–22.

81. Vaupel P, Kallinowski F, Okunieff P. Blood flow, oxygen and nutrient supply, and metabolic microenvironment of human tumors: a review. Cancer Res 1989;49(23):6449–65.

82. Zaca D, Hua J, Pillai JJ. Cerebrovascular reactivity mapping for brain tumor presurgical planning. World J Clin Oncol 2011;2(7):289–98.

83. Hsu YY, Chang CN, Jung SM, et al. Blood oxygenation level-dependent MRI of cerebral gliomas during breath holding. J Magn Reson Imaging 2004; 19(2):160–7.

84. Thomason ME, Burrows BE, Gabrieli JD, et al. Breath holding reveals differences in fMRI BOLD signal in children and adults. Neuroimage 2005; 25(3):824–37.

85. Magon S, Basso G, Farace P, et al. Reproducibility of BOLD signal change induced by breath holding. Neuroimage 2009;45(3):702–12.

86. Parkes MJ. Breath-holding and its breakpoint. Exp Physiol 2006;91(1):1–15.

87. Moreton FC, Dani KA, Goutcher C, et al. Respiratory challenge MRI: practical aspects. Neuroimage Clin 2016;11:667–77, 2213-1582 (Electronic).

88. Li TQ, Kastrup A, Takahashi AM, et al. Functional MRI of human brain during breath holding by BOLD and FAIR techniques. Neuroimage 1999; 9(2):243–9.

89. Kastrup A, Li TQ, Glover GH, et al. Cerebral blood flow-related signal changes during breath-holding. AJNR Am J Neuroradiol 1999;20(7):1233–8.

90. Bright MG, Bulte DP, Jezzard P, et al. Characterization of regional heterogeneity in cerebrovascular reactivity dynamics using novel hypocapnia task and BOLD fMRI. Neuroimage 2009;48(1):166–75.

91. van Niftrik CH, Piccirelli M, Bozinov O, et al. Fine tuning breath-hold-based cerebrovascular reactivity analysis models. Brain Behav 2016;6(2): e00426.

92. Birn RM, Smith MA, Jones TB, et al. The respiration response function: the temporal dynamics of fMRI signal fluctuations related to changes in respiration. Neuroimage 2008;40(2):644–54.

93. Kannurpatti SS, Biswal BB. Detection and scaling of task-induced fMRI-BOLD response using resting state fluctuations. Neuroimage 2008;40(4):1567–74.

94. Kannurpatti SS, Motes MA, Biswal BB, et al. Assessment of unconstrained cerebrovascular reactivity marker for large age-range FMRI studies. PLoS One 2014;9(2):e88751.

95. Kannurpatti SS, Motes MA, Rypma B, et al. Increasing measurement accuracy of age-related BOLD signal change: minimizing vascular contributions by resting-state-fluctuation-of-amplitude scaling. Hum Brain Mapp 2011;32(7):1125–40.

96. Wise RG, Ide K, Poulin MJ, et al. Resting fluctuations in arterial carbon dioxide induce significant low frequency variations in BOLD signal. Neuroimage 2004;21(4):1652–64.

97. Liu PY, Li Y, Pinho M, et al. Cerebrovascular reactivity mapping without gas challenges. Neuroimage 2017;146:320–6, 1095-9572 (Electronic).

98. Ghinda DC, Wu JS, Duncan NW, et al. How much is enough—can resting state fMRI provide a demarcation for neurosurgical resection in glioma? Neurosci Biobehav Rev 2018;84:245–61, 1873-7528 (Electronic).

99. Zaca D, Corsini F, Rozzanigo U, et al. Whole-brain network connectivity underlying the human speech articulation as emerged integrating direct electric stimulation, resting state fMRI and tractography. Front Hum Neurosci 2018;12:405, 1662-5161 (Print).

100. Qiu TM, Gong FY, Gong X, et al. Real-time motor cortex mapping for the safe resection of glioma: an intraoperative resting-state fMRI study. AJNR Am J Neuroradiol 2017;38(11):2146–52.

101. Zaca D, Jovicich J, Corsini F, et al. ReStNeuMap: a tool for automatic extraction of resting-state functional MRI networks in neurosurgical practice. J Neurosurg 2018;131(3):764–71.

102. Yahyavi-Firouz-Abadi N, Pillai JJ, Lindquist MA, et al. Presurgical brain mapping of the ventral somatomotor network in patients with brain tumors using resting-state fMRI. Am J Neuroradiol 2017; 38(5):1006–12.

103. Wongsripuemtet J, Tyan AE, Carass A, et al. Preoperative mapping of the supplementary motor area in patients with brain tumor using resting-state fMRI with seed-based analysis. Am J Neuroradiol 2018;39(8):1493–8.

104. Voets N, Plaha P, Parker Jones O, et al. Presurgical localization of the primary sensorimotor cortex in gliomas : when is resting state FMRI beneficial and sufficient? Clin Neuroradiol 2020. https://doi.org/10.1007/s00062-020-00879-1.

105. Dierker D, Roland JL, Kamran M, et al. Resting-state functional magnetic resonance imaging in presurgical functional mapping: sensorimotor localization. Neuroimaging Clin N Am 2017;27(4): 621–33.

106. Vakamudi K, Posse S, Jung R, et al. Real-time presurgical resting-state fMRI in patients with brain tumors: Quality control and comparison with task-fMRI and intraoperative mapping. Hum Brain Mapp 2020;41(3):797–814.

107. Shimony JS, Zhang DY, Johnston JM, et al. Resting-state spontaneous fluctuations in brain activity; a new paradigm for presurgical planning using fMRI. Acad Radiol 2009;16(5):578–83.

108. Schneider FC, Pailler M, Faillenot I, et al. Presurgical assessment of the sensorimotor cortex using resting-state fMRI. Am J Neuroradiol 2016;37(1): 101–7.

109. Sair HI, Yahyavi-Firouz-Abadi N, Calhoun VD, et al. Presurgical brain mapping of the language network in patients with brain tumors using resting-state fMRI: Comparison with task fMRI. Hum Brain Mapp 2016;37(3):913–23.

110. Liu HS, Buckner RL, Talukdar T, et al. Task-free presurgical mapping using functional magnetic resonance imaging intrinsic activity Laboratory investigation. J Neurosurg 2009;111(4):746–54.

111. Agarwal S, Lu H, Pillai JJ. Value of frequency domain resting-state functional magnetic resonance imaging metrics amplitude of low-frequency fluctuation and fractional amplitude of low-frequency fluctuation in the assessment of brain tumor-induced neurovascular uncoupling. Brain Connect 2017;7(6):382–9.

112. Agarwal S, Sair HI, Gujar S, et al. Functional magnetic resonance imaging activation optimization in the setting of brain tumor-induced neurovascular uncoupling using resting-state blood oxygen level-dependent amplitude of low frequency fluctuations. Brain Connect 2019;9(3):241–50.

113. Agarwal S, Sair HI, Pillai JJ. The resting-state functional magnetic resonance imaging regional homogeneity metrics-Kendall's coefficient of concordance-regional homogeneity and coherence-regional homogeneity-are valid indicators of tumor-related neurovascular uncoupling. Brain Connect 2017;7(4):228–35.

114. Metwali H, Raemaekers M, Ibrahim T, et al. Inter-network functional connectivity changes in patients with brain tumors: a resting-state functional magnetic resonance imaging study. World Neurosurg 2020;138:e66–71, 1878-8769 (Electronic).

115. Liouta E, Katsaros VK, Stranjalis G, et al. Motor and language deficits correlate with resting state functional magnetic resonance imaging networks in patients with brain tumors. J Neuroradiol 2019;46(3): 199–206.

116. Mallela AN, Peck KK, Petrovich-Brennan NM, et al. Altered resting-state functional connectivity in the hand motor network in glioma patients. Brain Connect 2016;6(8):587–95.

117. Hadjiabadi DH, Pung L, Zhang J, et al. Brain tumors disrupt the resting-state connectome. Neuroimage Clin 2018;18:279–89, 2213-1582 (Electronic).

118. Lee MH, Miller-Thomas MM, Benzinger TL, et al. Clinical resting-state fMRI in the preoperative setting: are we ready for prime time? Top Magn Reson Imaging 2016;25:11–8, 1536-1004 (Electronic).

119. Zhang DY, Johnston JM, Fox MD, et al. Preoperative sensorimotor mapping in brain tumor patients using spontaneous fluctuations in neuronal activity imaged with functional magnetic resonance

imaging: initial experience. Neurosurgery 2009; 65(6):226–36.

120. Kokkonen SM, Nikkinen J, Remes J, et al. Preoperative localization of the sensorimotor area using independent component analysis of resting-state fMRI. Magn Reson Imaging 2009;27(6):733–40.

121. Mitchell TJ, Hacker CD, Breshears JD, et al. A novel data-driven approach to preoperative mapping of functional cortex using resting-state functional magnetic resonance imaging. Neurosurgery 2013;73(6):969–82.

122. Sair HI, Agarwal S, Pillai JJ. Application of resting state functional MR imaging to presurgical mapping: language mapping. Neuroimaging Clin N Am 2017;27(4):635–44.

123. Agarwal S, Sair HI, Pillai JJ. Limitations of resting-state functional MR imaging in the setting of focal brain lesions. Neuroimaging Clin N Am 2017; 27(4):645–61.

124. Waheed SH, Mirbagheri S, Agarwal S, et al. Reporting of resting-state functional magnetic resonance imaging preprocessing methodologies. Brain Connect 2016;6(9):663–8.

125. Fox MD, Corbetta M, Snyder AZ, et al. Spontaneous neuronal activity distinguishes human dorsal and ventral attention systems. Proc Natl Acad Sci U S A 2006;103(26):10046–51.

126. Vincent JL, Kahn I, Snyder AZ, et al. Evidence for a frontoparietal control system revealed by intrinsic functional connectivity. J Neurophysiol 2008; 100(6):3328–42.

127. Beckmann CF, DeLuca M, Devlin JT, et al. Investigations into resting-state connectivity using independent component analysis. Philos Trans R Soc Lond B Biol Sci 2005;360(1457):1001–13.

128. Damoiseaux JS, Rombouts SA, Barkhof F, et al. Consistent resting-state networks across healthy subjects. Proc Natl Acad Sci U S A 2006;103(37): 13848–53.

129. Lemee JM, Berro DH, Bernard F, et al. Resting-state functional magnetic resonance imaging versus task-based activity for language mapping and correlation with perioperative cortical mapping. Brain Behav 2019;9(10):e01362.

130. Bathla G, Gene MN, Peck KK, et al. Resting state functional connectivity of the supplementary motor area to motor and language networks in patients with brain tumors. J Neuroimaging 2019;29(4): 521–6.

131. Zang YF, Jiang TZ, Lu YL, et al. Regional homogeneity approach to fMRI data analysis. Neuroimage 2004;22(1):394–400.

132. Zang YF, He Y, Zhu CZ, et al. Altered baseline brain activity in children with ADHD revealed by resting-state functional MRI. Brain Dev 2007;29(2):83–91.

133. Biswal BB, Kannurpatti SS, Rypma B. Hemodynamic scaling of fMRI-BOLD signal: validation of low-frequency spectral amplitude as a scalability factor. Magn Reson Imaging 2007;25(10):1358–69.

134. Pronin IN, Batalov AI, Zakharova NE, et al. Evaluation of vascular reactivity to overcome limitations of neurovascular uncoupling in BOLD fMRI of malignant brain tumors. Zh Vopr Neirokhir Im N N Burdenko 2018;82(5):21–9 [in Russian].

135. Voss HU, Peck KK, Petrovich Brennan NM, et al. A vascular-task response dependency and its application in functional imaging of brain tumors. J Neurosci Methods 2019;322:10–22. https://doi.org/10.1016/j.jneumeth.2019.04.004.

Resting State Functional MR Imaging of Language Function

John J. Lee, MD, PhD[a], Patrick Luckett, PhD[b], Mohammad M. Fakhri, MD[a],
Eric C. Leuthardt, MD[c], Joshua S. Shimony, MD, PhD[a],*

KEYWORDS

- Language • Presurgical planning • Task fMRI • Resting state fMRI • FreeSurfer • Neurosynth
- Deep learning • Convolutional neural network

KEY POINTS

- Task functional MR imaging is the standard of care for mapping the language system before surgery.
- The language system is composed of multiple components and more than one task is typically required to fully localize the language system.
- Resting state functional MR imaging can localize the language system but its relationship to task functional MR imaging and anatomic landmarks has not been fully characterized.

INTRODUCTION

Localization of language regions using task-based functional MR imaging (T-fMR imaging) is currently considered standard of care before surgical resection of brain lesions that may impinge on these critical areas of the brain ("eloquent cortex").[1] This information is considered critical for presurgical planning, assessing the risk for morbidity, and consultation with patients and their families. This method is most often used for brain tumor resection, but has become common in numerous other neurosurgical procedures such as epilepsy surgery, brain biopsies, and laser ablation procedures.

Mapping language function accurately is complicated by several factors such as the numerous components of the language system (receptive vs expressive language, memory, reading, listening, and speaking that involve components of vision, hearing, and the motor systems),[2] and the variability of its location across patients even after hemispheric dominance is established. Further complicating the surgical plan is the need to integrate this information between aggressive resection (that can extend life and delay recurrence) and functional preservation (decreasing morbidity),[3–5] which can differ depending on the exact location of the tumor with respect to different parts of the language system. Some areas of the language system will not recover from resection (eg, Broca's area), but others may be fully restored after recovery time and therapy (eg, supplementary motor area).[6]

Although no one task can fully characterize the entire language system, a large collection of tasks have been developed as part of research in the field of system neurosciences.[7–9] These tasks have been designed to activate and map different components of the language system. Owing to

[a] Mallinckrodt Institute of Radiology, Washington University, 4525 Scott Avenue, St Louis, MO 63110, USA;
[b] Department of Neurology, Washington University School of Medicine, 4525 Scott Avenue, St Louis, MO 63110, USA; [c] Department of Neurological Surgery, Washington University School of Medicine, 4525 Scott Avenue, St Louis, MO 63110, USA
* Corresponding author. Washington University School of Medicine, 4525 Scott Avenue, Campus Box 8131, St Louis, MO 63110.
E-mail address: shimonyj@wustl.edu

Neuroimag Clin N Am 31 (2021) 69–79
https://doi.org/10.1016/j.nic.2020.09.005
1052-5149/21/© 2020 Elsevier Inc. All rights reserved.

time and patient participation constraints, it is necessary to customize the T-fMR imaging examination to the individual patient. The complexity of this task has not gone unnoticed in the research literature,[2,7,8,10] including a white paper from the American Society for Functional Neuroradiology.[9]

The need for patient participation in the task is critical for accurate language mapping. Alternative approaches are needed when a patient cannot participate in the task, such as in cases of confusion, disability, need for sedation, or in young children. One approach that is used by a several sites in such situations is resting state fMR imaging (RS-fMR imaging). Specifically, the multilayer perceptron algorithm[11] has been used successfully for language localization in a large series of patients.[12] This approach does not require patient participation and is able to extract language (and other) maps from calculations of functional connectivity across the brain.[13] Although further studies are needed to fully characterize the accuracy and usefulness of this method in surgery, preliminary studies indicate that it provides a fairly balanced map of the language system[14] and this result would be expected because it is not specific to any one task.

Customization of the T-fMR imaging study should take into account the condition of the patient (their ability to participate in the examination and how long they can lay still in the MR imaging scanner), the location of the tumor with respect to the language system, and the information that can be obtained from different specific language tasks. Several articles[2,7,8,10] have emphasized the need to map multiple language areas for surgical planning. The American Society for Functional Neuroradiology white paper is valuable in providing practical suggestions for task selection.[9]

Several recent technical developments in informatics techniques applied to neuroimaging analysis can help us quantitatively answer the central question of this study: How do the methods of T-fMR imaging and RS-fMR imaging compare in regard to localization of the language system? The tools used in this article include parcellations derived from the MNI152 atlas[15] using FreeSurfer[16] (surfer.nmr.mgh.harvard.edu), which has significantly improved our ability to characterize anatomic regions across the brain. The second tool used is the Neurosynth software platform[17] (www.neurosynth.org), which provides activation maps from meta-analysis of thousands of T-fMR imaging studies. The third tool we use is a deep learning 3-dimensional convolutional neural network (3D CNN), trained on thousands of normal subjects, which maps the language system using RS-fMR imaging.

METHODS
Anatomic Parcellation

Anatomic parcellation makes inferences based on neuroanatomy represented on the Montreal Neurologic Institute atlas, which includes the average of 152 T1-weighted MR imaging scans nonlinearly transformed into Talairach space (MNI152).[15] We applied the recon-all command from FreeSurfer on the MNI152 atlas to generate parcellations. We used FreeSurfer version 6.0.0. For this work, we curated FreeSurfer parcellations to coincide with 10 language-relevant anatomic regions described by Brennan and colleagues.[10] These regions can be roughly divided into 3 groups, from the frontal lobe, the parietal lobe, and the temporal lobe. From the frontal lobe, we defined Broca's area to comprise the left hemispheric pars opercularis and pars triangularis (FreeSurfer 1018, 1020). The dorsolateral prefrontal cortex (DLPFC) was manually curated by the union of the posterior portion of the rostral middle frontal region (FreeSurfer 1027, 2027), and the caudal middle frontal region (FreeSurfer 1003, 2003). The anterior insula was defined by FreeSurfer indices 1035, 2035, and the supplemental motor area was manually created from the portion of the superior frontal gyrus (FreeSurfer 1028, 2028) obliquely posterior to the RAS coordinate (−18.73, 27.58, 60.63). From the parietal lobe, the angular gyrus and supramarginal gyrus retained parcellations natively defined by FreeSurfer indices 11,125, 12,125, 1031, and 2031, respectively. From the temporal lobe, Wernicke's area was manually created from the superior temporal gyrus posterior to Heschl's gyrus. Heschl's gyrus, the middle temporal gyrus and inferior temporal gyrus retained parcellations natively defined by FreeSurfer indices 1034, 2034,1015, 2015, 1009, and 1009, respectively.

Task Functional MR Imaging Meta-Analysis

The Neurosynth software platform provides automations for parsing the texts of published task fMR imaging (T-fMR imaging) studies, identifying topical words that convey neuroimaging semantics, generating models for documents and their texts, parsing published tables for purposes of extracting task activation coordinates, and aggregating task activation data into visualizable statistical maps of significance. The developers of Neurosynth[17] were motivated by the need to aggregate and synthesize large numbers of T-fMR imaging studies disseminated across peer-reviewed publications. Because T-fMR imaging studies are often underpowered and have high false-positive rates, meta-analyses are useful for obtaining consistent, replicable quantitation with high specificity.[18,19] We used Neurosynth to generate automated meta-analyses that mapped a set of cognitive terms, curated from the literature,[8–10] to task activation maps.

Neurosynth extends the methods of information retrieval,[20] which have enabled modern Internet search engines, to support neuroimaging. We used Neurosynth's term frequency-inverse document frequency (tf-idf) scheme[20,21] to map terms to task activations. Queries of topical terms from a corpus of documents require scoring schemes for accurate query matches. Term frequency is the number of occurrences of a query term per document, evaluated over all documents. Inverse document frequency is $log(N/df)$ for N documents and df defined to be the number of documents containing a query term. Inverse document frequency assigns lower scores to query terms having little specificity (eg, "fMR imaging" in the corpus of documents in Neurosynth has high frequency and low information). The product tf-idf improves specificity for query terms occurring many times in a small number of documents (eg, "syntactic" in Neurosynth documents). Neurosynth directly maps tf-idf scores to task activations using activation coordinates parsed from documents. Thereby, we used Neurosynth to generate statistical maps of z-scores for χ^2 tests of significance on terms mapped to task activation coordinates. We used Neurosynth versions deployed at the web portal www.neurosynth.org in the spring of 2020. The active dataset for search queries was version 0.7, released in July 2018. The tf-idf scheme had been applied to the texts of all abstracts from 14,371 peer-reviewed documents published between 2000 and 2018. The active dataset provided 1335 searchable terms and enabled searching 507,891 task activations. We visualized terms mapped to task activations using the hyperbolic tangent of z-scores, which formally yielded correlation coefficients.

Table 1 describes an initial list of topical terms curated from the enumerations of frontal, parietal and temporal foci of task functionality given by Brennan and colleagues,[10] Zacá and colleagues,[8] and Black and colleagues.[9] We pruned this initial list according to the number of studies and number of activations reported by Neurosynth. For similar terms, for example, "semantic," "semantic memory," "semantically," and "semantics," we selected the topical term with the greatest number of studies and the greatest number of activations. We removed terms with correlation maps that possessed sparse, small clusters. We pruned further after comparing to FreeSurfer regions and resting state networks (RSNs), retaining terms with larger Jaccard and boundary F1 (BF1) similarity measures. Our final selection retained 15 topical terms: "attention," "hearing," "language," "lexical," "listening," "naming," "nouns," "phonological," "reading," "semantically," "sentence," "speech perception," "syntactic," "verb," and "words."

Mapping Language with Deep Learning

Deep learning computational models learn detailed representations of complex data and have been highly successful in visual object recognition.[22] Deep learning models comprise simple nonlinear modules that are composed in layers and other organizing structures. Model parameters learn the features of data in hierarchical layers of abstractions, such that higher level layers amplify features that are discriminating and suppress features with irrelevant variations. Compared with other machine learning methods, deep learning requires minimal domain-specific engineering, building internal representations directly from large amounts of available data and making use of extensive training computations. Multilayer perceptrons have successfully classified RSNs from RS-fMR imaging.[11] We made full use of the benefits of deep learning by using a 3D CNN with 3 and 5 cubic convolutions, 49 layers, and 3 dense blocks in a densely connected architecture.[23] The 3D CNN was implemented in Matlab R2019b (www.mathworks.com).

The 3D CNN was trained to classify brain regions belonging to a priori assigned RSNs. Training made use of normal human RS-fMR imaging data (n = 2795) from the Harvard-MGH Brain Genomics Superstruct Project[24] as well as from additional studies in progress at Washington University. These are detailed in Table 2 and include the Alzheimer's Disease Research Center,[25] the Dominantly Inherited Alzheimer's Network,[26] and the HIV Program at the Division of Infectious Diseases.[27] Each subject had approximately 14 min of RS-fMR imaging data (gradient echo echoplanar imaging with 3000 m TR, 3 mm cubic field of view), which were denoised, motion corrected, low-pass filtered and adjusted with global signal regression using methods previously described.[28] RSNs were identified from 300 spherical regions of interest (ROI), which had previously been identified on a meta-analysis of T-fMR imaging.[29] The choice of ROIs is detailed in Gordon and colleagues.[30] From the 300 ROIs we extracted a subset belonging to 9 RSNs that are associated with the language system. These include the ventral attention network (VAN), cingulo-opercular network (CON), auditory network (AUD), default

Table 1
Selected Neurosynth language terms associated with fMRI tasks

Term	No. of Studies	No. of Activations	fMRI Tasks
Attention	1831	65,346	Nonspecific (weak activity)
Hearing	124	4393	Passive story listening
Language	1101	42,749	Sentence completion Antonym generation Rhyming
Lexical	331	14,271	Sentence completion Antonym generation Rhyming
Listening	250	9819	Passive story listening
Naming	179	7361	Silent word/verb generation Object/category naming Noun–verb association
Nouns	100	4434	Silent word/verb generation Object/category naming Noun–verb association
Phonological	377	17,844	Sentence completion Antonym generation Rhyming
Reading	521	21,842	Sentence completion Reading comprehension
Semantically	122	4241	Silent word/verb generation Object/category naming Noun–verb association
Sentence	307	11,204	Sentence completion Antonym generation Rhyming
Speech Perception	97	3178	Passive story listening
Syntactic	169	5369	Silent word/verb generation Object/category naming Noun–verb association
Verb	127	5079	Silent word/verb generation Object/category naming Noun–verb association
Words	948	38,353	Sentence completion Antonym generation Rhyming

mode network (DMN), parietal memory network, fronto-parietal network (FPN), salience network (SAL), dorsal attention network (DAN), and medial temporal network (MTL). Of note, the 300 ROI parcellation does not have a separate language network; however, it includes the language system as a major component of the VAN. For each of the RSNs, an output map from the 3D CNN estimated the probability that voxels belonged to the RSN. Multiple (n = 268,000) example sets were generated from the data and then divided into training (n = 187,600) and validation (n = 80,400) sets. Outputs of our 3D CNN were native to a standardized atlas customized for scanners and preprocessing workflows at our institution and we linearly transformed these outputs to MNI152.

Similarity Measures

The Jaccard index between binarized images is the intersection of voxels divided by their union. It is a popular and well-characterized measure of the similarity of semantic segmentations. However, measures of voxel overlap do not provide information about boundaries. Also, low values of the Jaccard index can be difficult to interpret as

Table 2
Data sources for training 3D CNN

	GSP	ADRC	DIAN	HIV Program
No.	1137	1289	336	775
Age[a]	21.4 ± 2.4	68.1 ± 7.9	40.9 ± 10.9	44.3 ± 16.3
Scanner	Trio	Trio/Biograph	Trio/Verio	Trio/Prisma
Voxel size, cubic mm	3.0	4.0	3.3	4.0
Flip angle in degrees	85	90	80	90
Repetition time, ms	3000	2200	3000	2200
No. of fMR imaging frames	248	328	140	328

Abbreviations: ADRC, Alzheimer's disease research center; DIAN, dominantly inherited Alzheimer's network; GSP, genetics superstruct project; HIV, human immunodeficiency.
[a] Values are mean ± standard deviation.

estimators of statistical significance for noisy imaging data.[31]

For assessing the similarity of semantic segmentations, we also used the BF1 contour matching score.[31,32] BF1 scores are the product of precision and recall for boundary classifications divided by their sum. Their associated classifiers are trained with supervision to assign posterior probabilities for boundaries using local and global imaging features, such as voxel intensities, their gradients and orientations, texture features extracted by filter banks, results from clustering operations, and objective functions such as χ^2 on combinations of features. Combinations of features provide higher level information for boundary inferences. Studies of psychological perception suggest that humans also use combinations of cues when assessing boundaries.[33] The combination of BF1 score and Jaccard index correlates well with human preferences in usage tests of semantic segmentation.[31]

This article provides both measures to conform to the need for combinations of measures in clinically relevant decision-making. We used implementations of the Jaccard index and BF1 score provided by Matlab R2019b (www.mathworks.com).

RESULTS

The MNI152 atlas provides anatomic structures that we used with FreeSurfer parcellations and segmentations and manual adjustments thereof. Our adjustments specified anatomy that is, most relevant to language as described by Brennan and colleagues[10] and Black and colleagues.[9]

Fig. 1 shows fusion images for the probability of RSNs (rainbow colored) and the correlations of task activations (see **Fig.** 1A, gray-scaled) combined and overlaying the MNI152 atlas. **Fig.** 1B–J

show voxels (rainbow colored) for 9 RSNs associated with the language system as defined by a 3D CNN model. For clarity, probabilities of less than 0.05 are not displayed. To emphasize language-relevant topographies, viewport coordinates depicted as green crosshairs are centered on large volumes of probability that overlap with the language system in the left hemisphere. **Fig.** 1 also shows voxels (gray-scaled) for task activations identified by maps of correlation from Neurosynth as informed by 15 language-relevant topical terms. In **Fig.** 1 the displayed correlation map (gray-scaled) for task activations is the weighted average of correlations across Neurosynth terms with weights arising from Jaccard indices between term maps and resting state maps. For example, in **Fig.** 1B for VAN, which has a large overlap with the language system, gray-scaled voxels represent task activations for 14 out of 15 Neurosynth terms. The Neurosynth term "attention" overlaps with the DAN, but is not represented in **Fig.** 1B because it has no Jaccard overlap with the VAN. For reference purposes, **Fig.** 1A for "Neurosynth" shows the weighted average of correlations across all 15 Neurosynth terms for language. To facilitate comparison, **Fig.** 1A and B have identical viewport coordinates centered on Wernicke's area of the left hemisphere.

Fig. 1C–D and F–I describe the AUD, FPN, CON, DMN, MTL, and SAL networks. Left lateralization of the language centers is represented by Neurosynth's meta-analysis maps. Lateralization of the language centers is only marginally evident in the probability maps from our 3D CNN.

Figs. 2 and 3 represent similarity measures as heat maps and in a numerical format. The indices have been multiplied by 100 and rounded to integers for clarity of display. **Fig.** 2 shows the Jaccard index describing overlap of imaging voxels and **Fig.** 3 shows the BF1 contour matching score

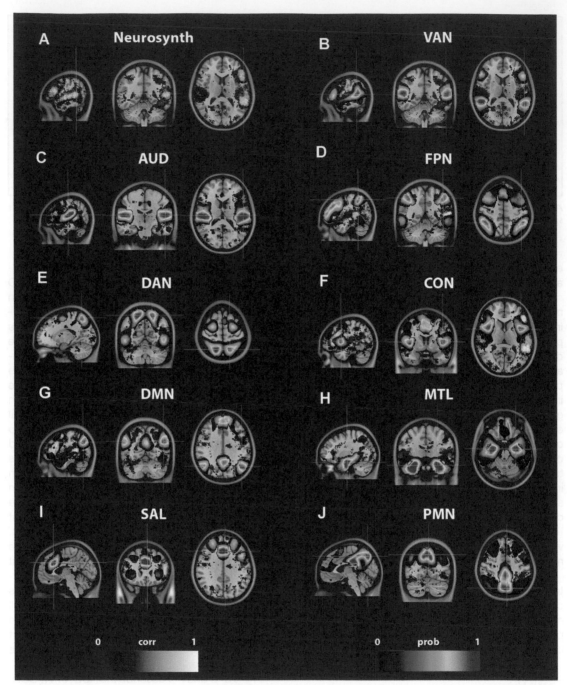

Fig. 1. Maps of the probability of RSNs (rainbow) and maps of correlations drawn from meta-analyses of task activations (*gray*-scaled) are superimposed on the Montreal Neurologic Institute atlas of 152 normal T1-weighted MR imaging scans (MNI152). A 3D CNN estimated the probability that voxels from resting state fMRI of normal subjects belonged to each of 9 classes of RSNs. Neurosynth provides correlations associated with tests of significance on meta-analyses of language-relevant topical terms. (*A*) Only Neurosynth correlations. (*B–J*) Fusions of RSNs and Neurosynth correlations in decreasing order of similarity.

describing boundary similarities. Qualitatively these 2 schemes give similar results, but the BF1 method demonstrated greater similarity of boundaries. These are each represented in 3 panels.

Panel (A) shows broad overlap of language task activations from Neurosynth with 3 important RSNs, the VAN, AUD, and FPN. Other networks, CON, DMN, and DAN, have smaller overlaps, but

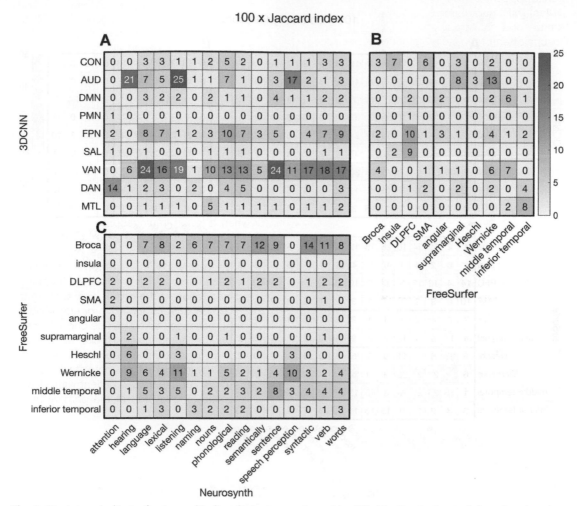

Fig. 2. Heatmaps indicate the Jaccard indices between anatomy identified by FreeSurfer, task functional regions identified by Neurosynth and RSNs identified by a deep 3D CNN. Between 2 binarized images, the Jaccard index is a segmentation measure that is, the intersection of voxels divided by the union of voxels. Jaccard indices have been multiplied by 100 and rounded to integers for clarity of display. (*A*) Comparing RSNs with Neurosynth. (*B*) Comparing FreeSurfer with RSNs. (*C*) Comparing Neurosynth with FreeSurfer. *Thickened lines* indicate the grouping of frontal, parietal, and temporal lobar anatomies. PMN, parietal memory network.

are widely spread over all activations. Not surprisingly, the DAN has larger overlap with tasks that require attention.

Panel (B) demonstrates overlap between Free-Surfer defined anatomic regions and RSNs. The VAN, FPN, CON, DAN, and DMN have broad overlap across many regions, however other RSNs are more specific. The SAL network is specific to the frontal regions (especially the DLPFC), MTL is specific to the temporal regions, and the AUD to the parietal area and Wernicke's area. Panel (C) may be the most useful for a practitioner showing the relationship between task activations from Neurosynth and anatomy from FreeSurfer. The dominance of Broca's, Wernicke's, and the middle temporal areas is clearly visualized. Additional

areas with weaker but widespread overlap with multiple tasks include the DLPFC and the other temporal lobe regions. One pattern that is evident in this panel is that some task terms are dominated by Wernicke's and the middle temporal gyrus (receptive language areas) (ie, hearing and speech perception), others are dominated by Broca's area (expressive language) (ie, semantically and naming), and many are more evenly balanced between the two (ie, language and lexical).

DISCUSSION

Localization of the language system for presurgical planning is complicated by the numerous components of the language system[2] and the variability

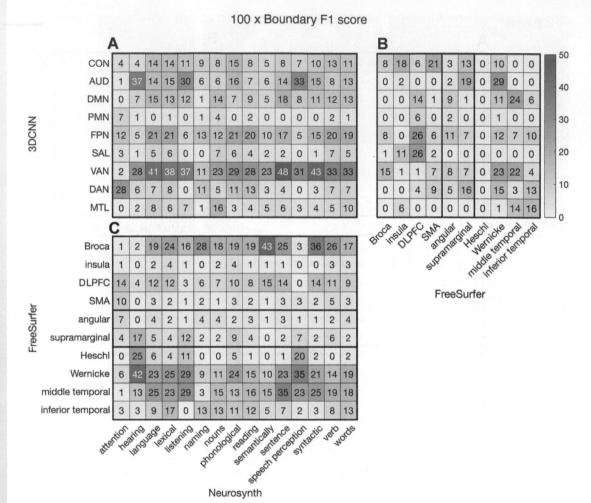

Fig. 3. Heatmaps indicate the BF1 contour matching score between anatomy revealed by FreeSurfer, task functional regions revealed by Neurosynth and RSNs revealed by a deep 3D CNN. BF1 is a semantic segmentation measure that emphasizes the similarity of boundaries between 2 binarized images, complementing the description of overlapping voxels provided by the Jaccard index. BF1 indices have been multiplied by 100 and rounded to integers for clarity of display. (*A*) Comparing RSNs with Neurosynth. (*B*) Comparing FreeSurfer with RSNs. (*C*) Comparing Neurosynth with FreeSurfer. Thickened lines indicate the grouping of frontal, parietal, and temporal lobar anatomies. PMN, parietal memory network.

of its location across patients.[34,35] The surgeon has to further take into account multiple factors such as the location and size of the tumor with respect to these different components, the condition and presenting symptoms of the patient, the expected aggressiveness of the tumor, and synthesize this information into a surgical plan, which may involve an awake craniotomy in some high-risk cases.

As the sophistication of fMR imaging techniques has increased, so have the demands for customized accurate language localization, using multiple T-fMR images to cover the full extent of the language network.[7–9] Distinctions between optimal tasks for adults and pediatric cases are also used to customize the T-fMR imaging protocol in

individuals.[9] The exact location and size of the tumor are also important factors in this ,process with an increased need for accuracy closer to the tumor.

Our goal in this article was to supplement the previously published guidelines for designing an optimal T-fMR imaging study with quantitative information obtained from large available data sets and new machine learning tools. Rutten and colleagues[7] demonstrated a high sensitivity for language localization as compared with intraoperative mapping using 4 tasks: verb generation, picture naming, verbal fluency, and sentence comprehension. Zacá and colleagues[8] concluded that silent word generation combined with a visual semantic paradigm (sentence completion or noun–verb association) sufficed to determine language localization and lateralization. Black and colleagues[9] present a white paper from the American Society for Functional Neuroradiology that recommended standardization of T-fMR imaging paradigms, processing and analysis across vendors and institutions. They propose separate tasks for adult and pediatric cases. For adults, they advocate the use of sentence completion, silent word generation, and one of the following: rhyming, object naming, or passive story listening.

For the purposes of building data-driven foundations, in **Table 1** we have paired paradigms from the literature with the large corpus of imaging data in Neurosynth, a meta-analysis framework driven by document models.

A comparison of the Neurosynth language terms with the Freesurfer regions provides insights into the subtle interactions of the language system across different activations. Tasks associated with semantics, naming, and syntax are strongly expressive and weighted toward Broca's area. In contrast, tasks associated with hearing, listening, and speech perception are strongly receptive and weighted toward Wernicke's area, Heschl's gyrus, and the middle temporal gyrus. The remaining task terms (such as lexical, language, phonology, reading, sentence, and words) are less specific and more balanced across the language areas. Similarly, anatomic regions, such as the DLPFC, supplemental motor area, and parietal areas are more balanced in their response across different task terms.

Current clinical use of RSNs for language localization is limited to a few sites despite the advantage of not requiring patient cooperation. The largest reported series of such clinical cases[12] has successfully used the multilayer perceptron algorithm[11] to localize RSNs. However, the association of the Neurosynth language terms with RSNs is instructive and could provide helpful information for future application using RSNs for presurgical language localization. Large overlaps are seen with various association networks, with special general language emphasis seen in the VAN and FPN, and a strong association of the receptive language terms with the AUD. Additional widespread associations are seen with the CON, DMN, and DAN, likely representing the need for engaging memory and attention functions as part of language activity.

Although the DAN overlaps with many areas engaged in various language tasks, it is highly focused with regard to attention-related task, likely indicating its engagement with the attentional aspects of language tasks.

A significant limitation of this study is the difficulty of mapping Neurosynth terms to task activations commonly reported in the neuroradiology literature. This difficulty reflects the limitations of the document models currently implemented by Neurosynth and elaborated in methods. Neurosynth maps language-relevant terms to absolute numbers of task activations in a statistically well-defined way (see **Table 1**). However, the detailed meaning of language-relevant terms is statistically averaged over documents accumulated in Neurosynth's document databases. For example, comparing the number of scans contributing to task inferences from Neurosynth and resting-state inferences from 3D CNN is not possible because Neurosynth's meta-analysis retains no structured information about scanning parameters or study protocols. Neurosynth provides only a count of terms in study documents and their tables of activation loci. At present, it is possible to make composite term queries from Neurosynth, such as "words and Broca" or "words and silent word generation" or "words and nouns and verb and association." However, logical intersections of terms produce much smaller samples of studies and activations. Consequently, sparse anatomic maps of task activations become vulnerable to underestimations of false discovery rates that Neurosynth parametrically applies to the entire corpus of documents in its databases. Additionally, the performance of Neurosynth on composite term queries is limited by its tf-idf document model, which is aware only of the presence of composite terms in a bag-of-words structure for any given document. The tf-idf models do not preserve the semantics of structured word combinations within documents.

SUMMARY

We provide quantitative information on the structure of the language system at the group level as determined using T-fMR imaging, RS-fMR imaging, and anatomic landmarks. Further work is needed at the individual level to help the practitioner better customize an optimal fMR imaging study to an individual patient and further the goal of precision medicine in presurgical planning.

ACKNOWLEDGMENTS

The authors thank the National Cancer Institute of the National Institute for Health for its support via grant R01CA203861.

DISCLOSURE

No conflicts for all authors.

REFERENCES

1. Petrella JR, Shah LM, Harris KM, et al. Preoperative functional MR imaging localization of language and motor areas: effect on therapeutic decision making in patients with potentially resectable brain tumors. Radiology 2006;240(3):793–802.
2. Benjamin CF, Walshaw PD, Hale K, et al. Presurgical language fMRI: mapping of six critical regions: fMRI mapping of six language-critical regions. Hum Brain Mapp 2017;38(8):4239–55.
3. McGirt MJ, Mukherjee D, Chaichana KL, et al. -Hinojosa A. Association of surgically acquired motor and language deficits on overall survival after resection of glioblastoma multiforme. Neurosurgery 2009; 65(3):463–70.
4. Lacroix M, Abi-Said D, Fourney DR, et al. A multivariate analysis of 416 patients with glioblastoma multiforme: prognosis, extent of resection, and survival. J Neurosurg 2001;95(2):190–8.
5. Gulati S, Jakola AS, Nerland US, et al. The risk of getting worse: surgically acquired deficits, perioperative complications, and functional outcomes after primary resection of glioblastoma. World Neurosurg 2011;76(6):572–9.
6. Vassal M, Charroud C, Deverdun J, et al. Recovery of functional connectivity of the sensorimotor network after surgery for diffuse low-grade gliomas involving the supplementary motor area. J Neurosurg 2017;126(4):1181–90.
7. Rutten GJM, Ramsey NF, Van Rijen PC, et al. Development of a functional magnetic resonance imaging protocol for intraoperative localization of critical temporoparietal language areas. Ann Neurol 2002; 51(3):350–60.
8. Zacà D, Jarso S, Pillai JJ. Role of semantic paradigms for optimization of language mapping in clinical fMRI studies. AJNR Am J Neuroradiol 2013; 34(10):1966–71.
9. Black DF, Vachha B, Mian A, et al. American society of functional neuroradiology–recommended fmri paradigm algorithms for presurgical language assessment. AJNR Am J Neuroradiol 2017;38(10): E65–73.
10. Brennan NP, Peck KK, Holodny A. Language mapping using fmri and direct cortical stimulation for brain tumor surgery: the good, the bad, and the questionable. Top Magn Reson Imaging 2016; 25(1):1–10.
11. Hacker CD, Laumann TO, Szrama NP, et al. Resting state network estimation in individual subjects. NeuroImage 2013;82:616–33.
12. Leuthardt EC, Guzman G, Bandt SK, et al. Integration of resting state functional MRI into clinical practice - A large single institution experience. PLOS ONE 2018;13(6):e0198349.
13. Dierker D, Roland JL, Kamran M, et al. Resting-state functional magnetic resonance imaging in presurgical functional mapping. Neuroimaging Clin N Am 2017;27(4):621–33.
14. Sair HI, Yahyavi-Firouz-Abadi N, Calhoun VD, et al. Presurgical brain mapping of the language network in patients with brain tumors using resting-state fMRI: comparison with task fMRI. Hum Brain Mapp 2016;37(3):913–23.
15. Grabner G, Janke AL, Budge MM, et al. Symmetric atlasing and model based segmentation: an application to the hippocampus in older adults. In: Larsen R, Nielsen M, Sporring J, editors. Medical image computing and computer-assisted intervention – MICCAI 2006. Lecture notes in computer science. Springer; 2006. p. 58–66. https://doi.org/10.1007/11866763_8.
16. Desikan RS, Ségonne F, Fischl B, et al. An automated labeling system for subdividing the human cerebral cortex on MRI scans into gyral based regions of interest. NeuroImage 2006;31(3):968–80.
17. Yarkoni T, Poldrack RA, Nichols TE, et al. Large-scale automated synthesis of human functional neuroimaging data. Nat Methods 2011;8(8):665–70.
18. Nielsen FÅ, Hansen LK, Balslev D. Mining for associations between text and brain activation in a functional neuroimaging database. Neuroinformatics 2004;2(4):369–79.
19. Wager TD, Lindquist MA, Nichols TE, et al. Evaluating the consistency and specificity of neuroimaging data using meta-analysis. NeuroImage 2009; 45(1, Supplement 1):S210–21.
20. Blei DM. Latent dirichlet allocation. J Mach Learn Res 2003;3(Jan):993–1022.
21. Manning C, Raghavan P, Schuetze H. Introduction to information retrieval. Cambridge University Press; 2008.
22. LeCun Y, Bengio Y, Hinton G. Deep learning. Nature 2015;521(7553):436.
23. Huang G, Liu Z, Pleiss G, et al. Convolutional networks with dense connectivity. IEEE Trans Pattern Anal Mach Intell 2019;1. https://doi.org/10.1109/TPAMI.2019.2918284. Published online.
24. Thomas Yeo BT, Krienen FM, Sepulcre J, et al. The organization of the human cerebral cortex estimated by intrinsic functional connectivity. J Neurophysiol 2011;106(3):1125–65.
25. Brier MR, Thomas JB, Snyder AZ, et al. Loss of intranetwork and internetwork resting state functional connections with Alzheimer's disease progression. J Neurosci 2012;32(26):8890–9.
26. Chhatwal JP, Schultz AP, Johnson KA, et al. Preferential degradation of cognitive networks differentiatoo Alzheimer's disease from ageing. Brain 2018; 141(5):1486–500.
27. Thomas JB, Brier MR, Snyder AZ, et al. Pathways to neurodegeneration: effects of HIV and aging on

resting-state functional connectivity. Neurology 2013;80(13):1186–93.

28. Power JD, Mitra A, Laumann TO, et al. Methods to detect, characterize, and remove motion artifact in resting state fMRI. NeuroImage 2014;84:320–41.

29. Power JD, Cohen AL, Nelson SM, et al. Functional network organization of the human brain. Neuron 2011;72(4):665–78.

30. Gordon EM, Laumann TO, Gilmore AW, et al. Precision functional mapping of individual human brains. Neuron 2017;95(4):791–807.e7.

31. Csurka G, Larlus D, Perronnin F. What is a good evaluation measure for semantic segmentation? In: Proceedings of the British machine vision conference 2013. British Machine Vision Association.

Durham (UK): Durham University; 2013. p. 32. 1–32.11. https://doi.org/10.5244/C.27.32.

32. Martin DR, Fowlkes CC, Malik J. Learning to detect natural image boundaries using local brightness, color, and texture cues. IEEE Trans Pattern Anal Mach Intell 2004;26(5):530–49.

33. Rivest J, Cabanagh P. Localizing contours defined by more than one attribute. Vision Res 1996;36(1): 53–66.

34. Sanai N, Mirzadeh Z, Berger MS. Functional outcome after language mapping for glioma resection. N Engl J Med 2008;358(1):18–27.

35. Agarwal S, Hua J, Sair HI, et al. Repeatability of language fMRI lateralization and localization metrics in brain tumor patients. Hum Brain Mapp 2018;39(12): 4733–42.

Dynamic Brain Connectivity in Resting State Functional MR Imaging

Rozita Jalilianhasanpour, MD[a], Daniel Ryan, MD[a], Shruti Agarwal, PhD[a],
Elham Beheshtian, MD[a], Sachin K. Gujar, MBBS[a], Jay J. Pillai, MD[a,b],
Haris I. Sair, MD[a,c],*

KEYWORDS

- Dynamic connectivity • Resting state MR imaging • Functional connectivity • Rs-fMRI
- Brain mapping

KEY POINTS

- Dynamic functional connectivity in resting state functional MR imaging may provide information that cannot be determined with traditional connectivity analysis.
- Dynamic functional connectivity correlates with different brain physiologic states and alterations of dynamic functional connectivity have been seen in various brain pathologies.
- Because resting state function MR imaging is increasingly being used in preoperative brain mapping, dynamic functional connectivity may be useful as an additional tool in this clinical setting.

DYNAMIC RESTING STATE FUNCTIONAL MR IMAGING

Resting state function MR imaging (rs-fMR imaging) demonstrates collections of distinct brain regions that exhibit low-frequency, temporally correlated blood oxygen level–dependent (BOLD) signal fluctuations in the absence of an explicit task, which are referred as resting-state networks.[1] With rs-fMR imaging, the anatomic understanding of brain function has evolved from a localizationist perspective to a network-based structure.[2] These networks tend to involve regions that are coactivated and observed with consistency across subjects and scanning periods, suggesting a general principle of brain functional organization. Currently, the analysis of resting-state networks typically uses techniques that assume temporal stationarity and measures of linear dependence are computed over the entire scan to characterize the strength of connections across regions.[3–6]

Although evident in studies of higher temporal resolution such as electroencephalography or magnetoencephalography, the fluctuation of neurophysiologic processes was initially excluded from consideration when analyzing rs-fMR imaging data, which assumed stationarity across the time of acquisition. However, increasingly, time varying changes in network connectivity, or dynamic functional connectivity (dFC) have been seen across different physiologic or pathologic brain conditions.[7–14] Additionally, evidence shows that inter-regional correlations can be modulated by cognitive processes that occur on time courses of a typical scan.[15] The "resting state" is a condition of undirected wakefulness that may encompass varying levels of attention, mind wandering, and arousal superimposed on fluctuating patterns

[a] Division of Neuroradiology, The Russell H. Morgan Department of Radiology and Radiological Science, Johns Hopkins University School of Medicine, 600 North Wolfe Street, Baltimore, MD 21287, USA; [b] Department of Neurosurgery, Johns Hopkins University School of Medicine, 1800 Orleans Street, Baltimore, MD 21287, USA; [c] The Malone Center for Engineering in Healthcare, The Whiting School of Engineering, Johns Hopkins University, Baltimore, MD, USA
* Corresponding author. Division of Neuroradiology, The Russell H. Morgan Department of Radiology and Radiological Science, Johns Hopkins University School of Medicine, 600 North Wolfe Street, Baltimore, MD 21287.
E-mail address: hsair1@jhmi.edu

Neuroimag Clin N Am 31 (2021) 81–92
https://doi.org/10.1016/j.nic.2020.09.004

of intrinsic brain function.[15] Studies suggest that dFC is in fact able to capture the alterations of intrinsic FC in various physiologic brain states and might be indeed a more sensitive marker than static FC.[16,17] In recent years, several studies have also discovered abnormal patterns of brain dFC (characterized by excessive of variability or stability over time) in schizophrenia, autism, dementia, multiple sclerosis, and depression disorders.[8–12,14,18] In fact, other brain conditions in which excessive variability or stability of thought processes could occur at different times also appear as ideal candidates to benefit from dFC research.[16]

In this article, we briefly review the underlying principles of dFC, examine techniques for assessing dFC in rs-fMR imaging and highlight selected patterns that emerge, and discuss potential clinical applications of dFC. Our goal is not to attempt a comprehensive review, for which there are many other resources available, but rather to provide a broad overview from which the interested reader can further add to their knowledge from the literature.

INTRINSIC CORRELATIONS OF THE BRAIN AND RELEVANCE TO DYNAMIC CONNECTIVITY

The mainstay of rs-fMR imaging analysis is to examine time-varying BOLD signal changes across brain regions while the subject is at rest, often with simple measures such as calculation of the Pearson correlation coefficient (**Fig. 1**). A collection of similarly time-varying regions is considered to represent intrinsic brain networks.[19,20] However, one must understand that the distinction between networks is not as clear-cut as expected. Although it is convenient to lump brain regions into different categories, the designation of brain networks is, to a certain extent, arbitrary.[16] For example, subcomponents of the default mode network (DMN) have been shown to demonstrate variable patterns of correlation and anticorrelation with distinct brain regions. Regions of anticorrelation using a seed in the anterior portion of the DMN, the ventromedial prefrontal cortex, comprised mainly of regions subserving visuospatial attention, whereas a seed in the posterior portion of the DMN, the posterior cingulate cortex, demonstrated anticorrelation with prefrontal planning and control circuits.[21] An interesting observation here is the distribution of primary anticorrelations with seed regions that are found toward the opposite parts of the brain. Therefore, subcomponents of what are often assumed to represent uniformly functioning networks (eg, the DMN), may in fact have different functional roles.

More interestingly, Chang and Glover[15] demonstrated that, when separately measuring correlations (in actuality, the anticorrelations) of the posterior cingulate gyrus in different time periods of rs-fMR imaging image acquisition, slightly different patterns of whole brain connectivity emerged, indicating nonstationarity in internetwork connectivity (**Fig. 2**).[15] The DMN is a network that is thought to be active in states of spontaneous mind wandering and in situations without

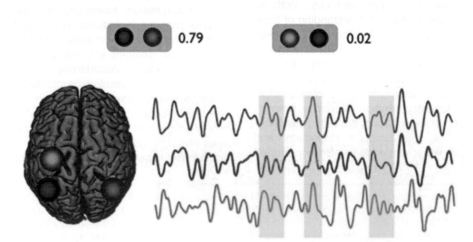

Fig. 1. BOLD time courses from 3 different seed regions of the brain in a single subject. Blue and red regions of interest (ROIs) reflect homotopic regions of the brain. In considering the total acquisition, BOLD signals of the blue and red ROIs are highly correlated (reflected by a Pearson coefficient of 0.79), and the BOLD signals of the green and red ROIs demonstrate essentially no correlation (Pearson coefficient of 0.02). However, when examining subsets of the waveforms, there are periods of transient synchrony across all 3 ROIs, shown in the *blue boxes.*

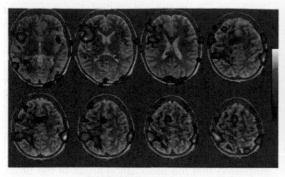 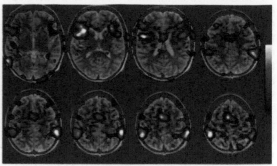

First 7 min   Second 7 min

Fig. 2. Negative correlations of a posterior cingulate seed region of interest across 2 successive 7-minute segments of resting-state data, shown for one subject. The distribution of anticorrelated networks is different between the 2 segments shown in the 2 separate panels, indicating time-varying correlations. (*From* Chang C, Glover GH. Time-frequency dynamics of resting-state brain connectivity measured with fMRI. Neuroimage. 2010;50(1):81-98. https://doi.org/10.1016/j.neuroimage.2009.12.011; with permission. Figure 14.)

a specific goal-directed behavior, generally demonstrating highly opposing patterns of correlations with the somatomotor network, a network that is functionally diametrically opposed to the DMN.[22] Although there have been discussions on whether this is an artifactual residue of processing methods that are beyond the scope of this review, the point still stands that there is a range of BOLD synchronicity across networks. An additional point that is often misunderstood is, in a sense, the equivalence of high correlations and high anticorrelations. In both situations, the fundamental process is a high level of interaction or communication. The lack of this communication or interaction would be manifest not as anticorrelation, but rather as no correlation.

The nature of dynamic correlations, or nonstationarity that is, supported by Chang and Glover's work,[15] can be illustrated by sampling representative seed regions of the DMN and somatomotor network (see **Fig. 2**). Here, time courses from 2 regions of the DMN (involving the inferior parietal lobules on each side) and 1 region of the somatomotor network (the precentral gyrus) are examined. As expected, homotopic regions of the brain (left and right inferior parietal lobules) demonstrate very high correlations across time, although there seems to be a low overall correlation between an inferior parietal lobule seed and the ipsilateral precentral gyrus seed. However, there do seem to be short instances of transient high correlations, or synchronicity, between them. Furthermore, when individual seed regions within networks are also examined, similar findings emerge, of a variable set of general strength of overall correlations between subcomponents of a network, however with instances of more

varying synchronicity, supporting both findings of Chang and Glover[15] (time-varying correlations) and Uddin and colleagues[21] (region-varying correlations).

GENERAL METHODS OF ASSESSING DYNAMIC FUNCTIONAL CONNECTIVITY

The general principle of dFC being the determination of assessment of time-varying changes in function, several methods of obtaining the data exist; the simplest to use is sliding time windows to summarize epochs of correlations. Connectivity can be computed between each pair of time courses as a Pearson correlation coefficient within a specified temporal window that is then shifted by a step, and the same calculations are repeated over the time interval. This process is repeated until the window reaches the end point of time courses, to ultimately obtain the time-varying connectivity time course. Values are generally summarized into a matrix describing the connectivity pattern of the brain during the examined temporal interval.[16,23–25]

An extension of this method to identify the source time courses is to use network-based connectivity parameters rather than that which is seed based or region based.[24,26] Independent component analysis (ICA) can be performed at a group level on a set of subjects to generate a map of consistent brain networks across the cohort.[27] The individual time courses now are generated from each individual ICA component that reflects the representative signal of each network or network subcomponent. Each individual's unique corresponding subnetwork is back reconstructed to obtain the individual subnetwork time courses, and a subnetwork versus subnetwork correlation matrix generated. A sliding window approach to these data then yields a set of time-varying connectivity matrices for each subject. Allen and colleagues[24] demonstrate that following clustering of these resultant dFC maps, a consistent set of "states" of connectivity can be seen (**Fig. 3**).[26] They extend the analysis to demonstrate limited sets of patterns of transitions that occur between the different states. Furthermore, when examining the range of variability of subnetworks across, time, an interesting property emerged (**Fig. 4**).[24] The different subnetworks exhibit different ranges of this variability, and mapping these regions coined the "zones of instability" to the brain demonstrate that the medial prefrontal cortex, the posterior cingulate cortex, and the inferior parietal lobules were the regions of the brain with the highest variability. All of these regions comprise subnetworks of the DMN. Of particular interest is the overlap between these brain regions of high variability or instability and the spatial distribution of brain regions that determine individuality (**Fig. 5**).[28] Here, Airan and colleagues[28] used an

unsupervised algorithm to pair together a set of unlabeled rs-fMR imaging from data that was comprised of test–retest rs-fMR imaging scans of healthy subjects. The algorithm was able to correctly pair the subjects' rs-fMR imaging scans with high accuracy; the regions of the brain that contributed most to the algorithm's ability to discriminate between subjects was then determined and was composed of the higher order association cortices, including regions associated with the DMN.[28] It is, at a fundamental level, not surprising that the association areas of the brain, which drive unique processes of the individual as opposed to more functionally homogenous regions such as the primary cortices (motor, visual, etc), also show a high degree of instability.

Exogenous agents can also modulate the dFC states. In a study examining the effect of isoflurane levels on dFC, increased levels were shown to result in increased "dwell times," or inertia, within a particular state, with decreased frequency of state-to-state transitions as well.[29] The overall number of individual states also decreased as the level of anesthesia increased. Indirectly, this

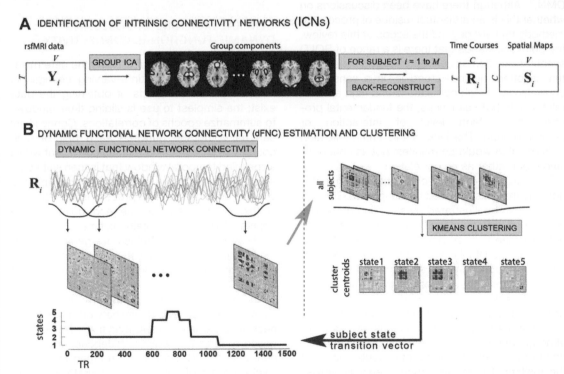

Fig. 3. Assessment of dFC incorporating group ICA to decompose fMR imaging data into intrinsic connectivity networks (*A*), with subsequent sliding window covariance estimation of the resultant network time courses (*B*), top left image labeled "ICN time courses". For each window, a correlation matrix is generated (*B*), lower panel labeled "dFNC windows", and the stack of matrices can then be clustered (in this case using k-means clustering (*B*), right panel) to identify states, and determine which state a given subject is occupying at a given time (*B*), left panel bottom, labeled "states". (*From* Damaraju E, Tagliazucchi E, Laufs H, Calhoun VD. Connectivity dynamics from wakefulness to sleep. Neuroimage. 2020 Jun 17;220:117047. https://doi.org/10.1016/j/neuroimage.2020.117047; with permission.)

Zones of Instability

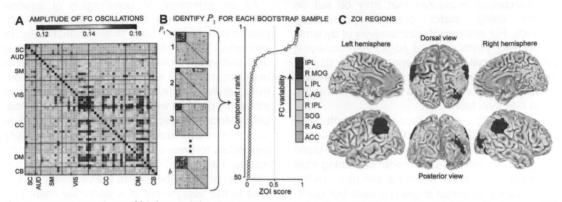

Fig. 4. Mapping regions of high variability in connectivity across time. (A) The amplitude of low-frequency oscillations between intrinsic brain networks, averaged across all subjects in the study, with greater amplitude indicating more variable functional connectivity. (B) Zones of instability (ZOI) scores are calculated using a bootstrap partitioning procedure. Networks with ZOI score of greater than 0.5 (regions of high variability in connectivity) are mapped onto surface rendered brain images (C). Note that these regions comprise major components of the DMN. (*From* Allen Elena A, Damaraju Eswar, Plis Sergey M, et al. Tracking whole-brain connectivity dynamics in the resting state. Cereb Cortex 2014;24(3):663–76; with permission.)

also supports the role of dynamic correlations in the manifestation of the "self" described elsewhere in this article.

More recently, the use of mind-altering agents (specifically hallucinogens) have been explored as a novel mechanism for conditions or situations that may be resistant to conventional methods of treatment. Psilocybin, for example, has been used in studies for intervention for smoking cessation or to treat depression.[30–33] Indeed, dynamic connectivity patterns are shown to be altered when psilocybin is administered; although the authors did not specifically correlate the dFC changes with behavioral measures, it would be interesting to see whether similar findings are manifest between the changes in dFC after psilocybin administration and behavioral measures.[34]

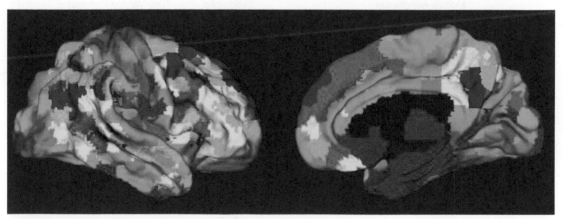

Fig. 5. Regions that most contribute to identification of the "individual" from rs-fMR imaging. Warmer colors indicate areas with high uniqueness across individuals (red being highest), and greater ability to discriminate between subjects, or in another sense, areas that determine individuality. Cooler colors indicate areas that are relatively consistent in connectivity pattern across subjects, thus contributing little to individual identification. As expected, association areas are more contributory to individuality. Of note, many of these regions comprise areas of the DMN, and have significant overlap with the ZOIs described in Fig. 4. (*Adapted from* Airan RD, Vogelstein JT, Pillai JJ, Caffo B, Pekar JJ, Sair HI. Factors affecting characterization and localization of interindividual differences in functional connectivity using MRI. Hum Brain Mapp. 2016;37(5):1986-1997. https://doi.org/10.1002/hbm.23150; with permission (Figure 5 in original).)

There are, however, other studies demonstrating a correlation of sliding window analyses with behavioral measures that may be not be evident using static connectivity analysis methods. For example, factor analysis of dynamic connectivity yields a set of edges with covarying connectivity that can be separated into defined groups. One specific factor of the dorsal attention network has been shown to predict performance on an attention task.[35]

More broadly, a study specifically contrasting static FC and dFC in mind wandering demonstrated that while there was no correlation of static FC measures with levels of mind-wandering after the administration of a painful stimulus, sliding window analysis in fact showed a weak but significant correlation with greater variability in connectivity measures correlating with higher rates of mind wandering and thoughts unrelated to the painful stimulus.[36] Conceivably, dFC measures such as this may be used in conjunction with neurofeedback mechanisms as a potential treatment for chronic pain syndromes.

As an extension to seed/region of interest (ROI)–based analysis, graph theoretic approaches have been used to summarize network properties of functional connectivity, including dFC analysis. Nodes represent subsegments of brain regions, and edges represent the connectivity between them. Network properties such as efficiency or small worldness can be easily calculated. Modularity represents the product of clustering of nodes that share similar connectivity properties to detect community structure in networks. Two complementing sets of properties can then be described. First, the variability across time in the assignment of a particular node to a specific module or community, and second, the variability of the strength of the patterns of edges that describe a particular module (**Fig. 6**).[37] Annotated graphs extend the ability to inform characteristics of graph components by incorporating

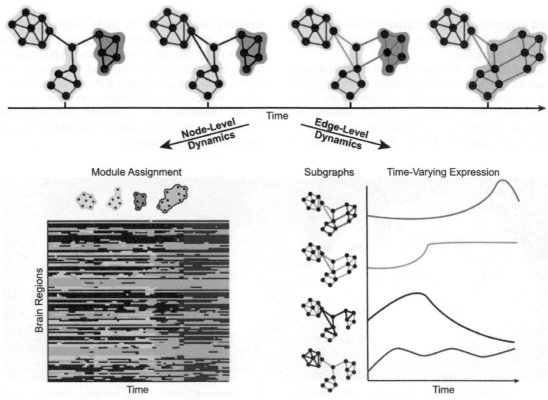

Fig. 6. Incorporating graph theory in dFC. Nodes are equivalent to seed regions or regions of interest from which time courses can be extracted. Edges represent the connectivity between node pairs. Strongly connected nodes constitute communities, or modules. Sets of edges that demonstrate similar strength or covariance across time are defined as subgraphs. Each unique color denotes a unique module or subgraph. Across time, a particular node can be part of a different module (*bottom left*), or a particular edge in a subgraph can have varying levels of strength, or expression (*bottom right*). (*From* Khambhati AN, Sizemore AE, Betzel RF, Bassett DS. Modeling and interpreting mesoscale network dynamics. Neuroimage. 2018;180(Pt B):337-349. https://doi.org/10.1016/j.neuroimage.2017.06.029; with permission.)

specific properties of the node itself to the overall graph structure. An example of intrinsic node properties would be, for example, the amplitude of BOLD activation for a region, as opposed to additional calculated graph metrics of a node such as node degree. By using annotated graphs, the discrepancy between BOLD magnitude of individual nodes (ie, the annotated nodes) and the community structure of the functional connectivity patterns (ie, the graph edges) was shown to predict individual differences in learning of a new motor skill.[38]

The assignment of node elements to community structure, or more precisely the change in module assignment over time, can in one sense be thought of as wandering, or in a more positive light, flexibility. Sliding window analyses with subsequent dynamic graph construction and calculation of this measure of flexibility (measured as the change in community assignment averaged over a set of predefined nodes) demonstrated that in patients with schizophrenia, there was a significant increase in flexibility of brain networks compared with healthy controls.[39] Furthermore, flexibility of first-degree relatives of patients with schizophrenia, but themselves without evidence of disease, was also significantly increased compared with healthy controls. Thus, dFC analyses may also aid in the stratification of at-risk individuals for various diseases. Finally, in the same investigation, the authors demonstrate that administering dextromethorphan, an NMDA antagonist, to healthy controls resulted in increased flexibility of networks compared with placebo. This finding supports the hypothesis of NMDA receptor hypofunction in schizophrenia.[40]

BEYOND CLASSIC SLIDING WINDOW ANALYSES

The major limitation in using any form of sliding window analysis is the a priori selection of the best window period for the analysis. To choose the best length, a trade-off must be reached for the optimal ranges of specificity (long enough to detect reliable dFC fluctuations) and sensitivity (short enough not to miss genuine dFC variations); however, it remains arbitrary and a matter of debate. Another limitation of sliding window analysis is the necessity of a fixed window length, thus limiting the analysis to the fluctuations in the frequency ranges within the window size, not the actual frequencies of the data, which may be more variable. One method to account for this is to calculate the similarity of the neural activation patterns in specific discrete time windows of varying widths.[41,42] Each time window represents a

node in the adjacency matrix, and the correlations computed across other nodes of time windows. Similar to Erhardt and Allen's findings, a set of consistent brain states emerge across time; in addition, varying time window lengths demonstrate different patterns of connectivity; as expected slow (longer) time scales showing a simpler, broader pattern, and fast (shorter) time scales showing more detailed variations in correlation.[37,41,43–45]

There are multiple other methods of countering this limitation of sliding window analysis. Time–frequency analysis, a modification of sliding window analysis, allows for temporal exploration of FC at multiple frequencies, adapting the observation window to the frequency content of the original time courses with adding an additional dimension to the parameter space.[15,29,46] Dynamic connectivity detection is another approach to replace the arbitrary parameter choice in the sliding window with a data-driven window selection.[29] This method allows the detection of time points when changes in FC occur and defines temporal windows for dFC analysis within these change points. Notably, a more recent similar approach has been developed in which an initially short window length is chosen, and then gradually increases until an assumption of local stationarity in the data becomes invalid. With this method, tailored windows with various sizes can span the whole time course of brain activity.[47]

Quasiperiodic pattern analysis (QPPA), a modification of sliding window analysis, has found to be relatively invariant in susceptibility to the choice of window length in some cases (**Fig. 7**).[48] In this method, a consecutive set of images is sampled and serves as a template. A sliding correlation is then computed between this template and the source data, yielding a waveform depicting the time-varying strength of similarity between the source data and the template. The images from the peaks of similarity are extracted and averaged to yield an updated template. This process is repeated until the template does not update for 2 successive iterations. As shown in **Fig. 7**, the choice of window length did not have a strong effect on the sliding correlations with the template. Similar findings have been shown in mice, rat, and human studies of QPPA.[48–52] Interestingly, some studies using QPPA show that the selection of the initial time frame to use as the template did not have an effect on the consistency of the final results, whereas other studies show that, in fact, this initial selection did contribute to differences in the results. The latter certainly makes sense when examining these findings in species with higher cognitive abilities such as humans, because

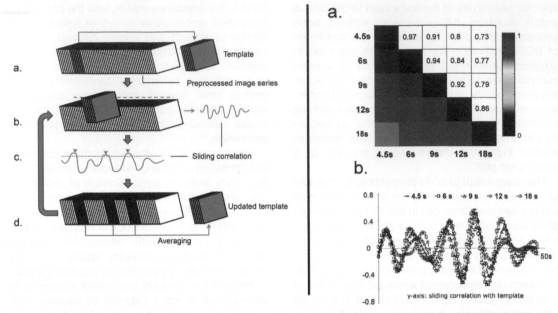

Fig. 7. Quasiperiodic pattern analysis. A consecutive set of images is initially sampled (*a, left*) and serves as a template. A sliding correlation is computed between the template and the source data (*b, left*). The segments that constitute the peaks of the correlations (*c* and *d, left*), are then averaged and incorporated into an updated template, and the above steps are repeated until stability of the template is demonstrated across 2 successive iterations. In this study, the choice of window length did not have a significant effect on the sliding correlations with the template (*a* and *b, right*). (*From* Majeed W, Magnuson M, Hasenkamp W, et al. Spatiotemporal dynamics of low frequency BOLD fluctuations in rats and humans. Neuroimage. 2011;54(2):1140-1150. https://doi.org/10.1016/j.neuroimage.2010.08.030.)

a higher frequency of neurocognitive changes and greater variability in differences between brain states are likely present across time. Despite this limitation, QPPA demonstrates a consistent pattern of propagation of network signals across the brain.

There are 2 other recent multivariate volatility models proposed for the study of dFC that refine the concept of sliding windows: dynamic conditional correlation (DCC) and exponentially weighted moving average, respectively.[53] These are parametric models for conditional covariance/correlation between time courses, which provide solutions for some of the limitations of sliding window approaches, such as noise susceptibility and suboptimal detection of subtle and/or abrupt changes in FC.[53,54] DCC in particular, has shown remarkable potential for effective estimation of dynamic changes in FC. Previous studies have shown that DCC is less susceptible to changes in FC induced by random noise. In addition, all the parameters in DCC model are calculated through quasimaximum likelihood methods which do not require a priori selections. In this model, dynamic variance/correlation are first calculated for each time courses, then the

standardized residuals are used to estimate dFC measures. A study by Lindquist and colleagues[53] compared the properties of DCC and other commonly used techniques in a series of simulation studies and reported that DCC demonstrated the optimal balance between sensitivity and specificity in detecting temporal changes in FC. The authors also highlighted that DCC provides a framework for statistical inference on dynamic variance and correlation, which is not available among other techniques. They therefore suggest that using a DCC approach would maximize the accuracy and reliability of dFC measures.

In another study, using test–retest rs-fMR imaging data on a cohort of healthy subjects and time courses derived from ICA component maps (similar to Erhardt and colleagues[26]), Choe and colleagues[55] found that, although DCC was comparable with sliding window analysis in estimating the means of dynamic correlations, it was also superior in estimating the reliability of variance across network pairs. An interesting and very practical byproduct of their analysis was that measuring the edge variance across ICA components was helpful in distinguishing between real intrinsic brain network

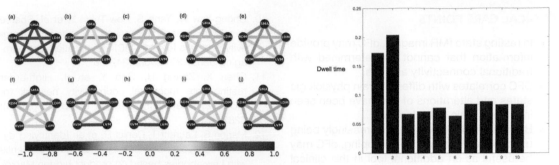

Fig. 8. The dFC of the somatomotor network (SMN). The network graphs on the left show 10 connectivity states that were found after clustering of time-varying matrices generated by DCC analysis. Bar graph on the right demonstrates the length of time, or dwell time, in a particular state across the scan length. The most prevalent state (state 2 in the figure) is a state of generally intermediate connectivity across the subsegments of the SMN. The state of high connectivity across the SMN (state 1) is the second most highest state, and is only seen in less than 20% of the total scan length. Additional intermediate states are evident and are fully described in Syed and colleagues (*From* Syed MF, Lindquist MA, Pillai JJ, et al. Dynamic Functional Connectivity States Between the Dorsal and Ventral Sensorimotor Networks Revealed by Dynamic Conditional Correlation Analysis of Resting-State Functional Magnetic Resonance Imaging. Brain Connect. 2017;7(10):635-642. https://doi.org/10.1089/brain.2017.0533; with permission.)

ICA components and noise components. Intrinsic networks demonstrated high variance between pairs of any network subcomponents, whereas noise components demonstrated consistently low variance, both to other noise components and to any network subcomponents. In this way, automated and reliable labeling of noise components in ICA may be possible, which is an important factor in adopting rs-fMR imaging as a translational tool.

Increasingly, rs-fMR imaging is being used as an adjunct to task-fMR imaging for presurgical brain mapping, and of all potential clinical applications, is the most promising as a tool for clinical practice.[56–59] However, the adoption of rs-fMR imaging in practice still has not become ubiquitous.[60] There are overlapping neurophysiologic considerations, such as neurovascular uncoupling in both rs-fMR imaging and task-fMR imaging.[61–64] A potential limiting factor of rs-fMR imaging is the subject-level variability of accuracy of rs-fMR imaging motor and language maps.[64–67] What could be the potential source of this variability? In examining the time-varying connectivity patterns of subcomponents of the motor network using DCC, Syed and colleagues[68] show that even within the subsystem of the motor network, there are a set of variables, however consistent, patterns or states of connectivity (**Fig. 8**). Of note, measurement of the dwell times of each state demonstrated that the most prevalent state (comprising approximately 20% of the total scan time) was not a state of high correlation between motor network subcomponents, but rather a "dormant" state with relatively low correlations (see

Fig. 8).[68] The state with high correlations within motor network components represented only the second most prevalent state of approximately 17% to 18%, and other variations of connectivity patterns comprised the rest. Given that the major contribution to motor network identification through seed-based methods or ICA would derive principally from the state with high within-network connectivity, this means that, in essence, less than 20% of the data during the time of acquisition actually contributed to target network identification. In other words, the engagement of specific brain network across time at rest may inform the likelihood of obtaining accurate network topology. DFC analysis of rs-fMR imaging data, therefore, may be used to improve reliability and accuracy of network characterization, a necessity for preoperative brain mapping.[66,68]

SUMMARY

Dynamic FC adds another dimension to rs-fMR imaging analysis, providing information on functional connectivity that cannot be determined using conventional static rs-fMR imaging analysis techniques. Consistent sets of brain states and spatial drift of functional connectivity can be found using dFC, and these measures correlate with different states of awareness or consciousness, and furthermore are shown to be altered in disease. Therefore, dFC may be a promising tool to add to the armamentarium of clinical functional neuroimaging, in particular in the setting of preoperative brain mapping, where rs-fMR imaging is already increasingly used.

CLINICAL CARE POINTS

- In resting state fMR imaging, dFC may provide information that cannot be determined with traditional connectivity analysis.
- DFC correlates with different brain physiologic states and alterations of dFC have been seen in various brain pathologies.
- Because rs-fMR imaging is increasingly being used in preoperative brain mapping, dFC may be useful as an additional tool in this clinical setting.

DISCLOSURE

The authors have nothing to disclose.

REFERENCES

1. Biswal B, Yetkin FZ, Haughton VM, et al. Functional connectivity in the motor cortex of resting human brain using echo-planar MRI. Magn Reson Med 1995;34(4):537–41.
2. Damoiseaux JS, Rombouts SARB, Barkhof F, et al. Consistent resting-state networks across healthy subjects. Proc Natl Acad Sci U S A 2006;103(37): 13848–53.
3. Greicius Michael D, Ben K, Reiss Allan L, et al. Functional connectivity in the resting brain: a network analysis of the default mode hypothesis. Proc Natl Acad Sci U S A 2003;100(1):253–8.
4. Beckmann Christian F, Marilena D, Devlin Joseph T, et al. Investigations into resting-state connectivity using independent component analysis. Philos Trans R Soc Lond B Biol Sci 2005;360(1457): 1001–13.
5. Raymond S, John S, Christian S, et al. Undirected graphs of frequency-dependent functional connectivity in whole brain networks. Philos Trans R Soc Lond B Biol Sci 2005;360(1457):937–46.
6. Aviv M, Yossi Y, Pasternak O, et al. Cluster analysis of resting-state fMRI time series. Neuroimage 2009; 45(4):1117–25.
7. Du Y, Pearlson Godfrey D, Yu Q, et al. Interaction among subsystems within default mode network diminished in schizophrenia patients: a dynamic connectivity approach. Schizophr Res 2016;170(1): 55–65.
8. Barnaly R, Eswar D, Pearlson Godfrey D, et al. Dynamic connectivity states estimated from resting fMRI Identify differences among Schizophrenia, bipolar disorder, and healthy control subjects. Front Hum Neurosci 2014;8:897.
9. Price T, Chong-Yaw W, Gao W, et al. Multiple-network classification of childhood autism using functional connectivity dynamics. Med Image Comput Comput Assist Interv 2014;17(Pt 3):177–84.
10. Chong-Yaw W, Yang S, Pew-Thian Y, et al. Sparse temporally dynamic resting-state functional connectivity networks for early MCI identification. Brain Imaging Behav 2016;10(2):342–56.
11. Chen X, Zhang H, Gao Y, et al. High-order resting-state functional connectivity network for MCI classification. Hum Brain Mapp 2016;37(9): 3282–96.
12. Marion S, Laurent T, Daniel R, et al. Identifying dynamic functional connectivity changes in dementia with Lewy bodies based on product hidden Markov models. Front Comput Neurosci 2016;10:60.
13. Nora L, Jonas R, Markus G, et al. Principal components of functional connectivity: a new approach to study dynamic brain connectivity during rest. Neuroimage 2013;83:937–50.
14. Kaiser Roselinde H, Whitfield-Gabrieli S, Dillon Daniel G, et al. Dynamic resting-state functional connectivity in major depression. Neuropsychopharmacology 2016;41(7):1822–30.
15. Chang C, Glover Gary H. Time-frequency dynamics of resting-state brain connectivity measured with fMRI. Neuroimage 2010;50(1):81–98.
16. Preti Maria G, Bolton Thomas Aw, Van De Ville D. The dynamic functional connectome: state-of-the-art and perspectives. Neuroimage 2017;160:41–54.
17. Lurie Daniel J, Daniel K, Bassett Danielle S, et al. Questions and controversies in the study of time-varying functional connectivity in resting fMRI. Netw Neurosci 2020;4(1):30–69.
18. Kalina C, Irving Zachary C, Fox Kieran CR, et al. Mind-wandering as spontaneous thought: a dynamic framework. Nat Rev Neurosci 2016;17(11): 718–31.
19. De Luca M, Beckmann CF, De Stefano N, et al. fMRI resting state networks define distinct modes of long-distance interactions in the human brain. Neuroimage 2006;29(4):1359–67.
20. Zarrar S, Clare KAM, Reiss Philip T, et al. The resting brain: unconstrained yet reliable. Cereb Cortex 2009;19(10):2209–29.
21. Uddin Lucina Q, Clare Kelly AM, Biswal Bharat B, et al. Functional connectivity of default mode network components: correlation, anticorrelation, and causality. Hum Brain Mapp 2009;30(2):625–37.
22. Vatansever D, Menon DK, Manktelow AE, et al. Default mode network connectivity during task execution. Neuroimage 2015;122:96–104.
23. Enzo T, von Wegner F, Astrid M, et al. Dynamic BOLD functional connectivity in humans and its electrophysiological correlates. Front Hum Neurosci 2012;6:339.
24. Allen Elena A, Eswar D, Plis Sergey M, et al. Tracking whole-brain connectivity dynamics in the resting state. Cereb Cortex 2014;24(3):663–76.
25. Pablo B, Lynn U, Sitt Jacobo D, et al. Signature of consciousness in the dynamics of resting-state brain

activity. Proc Natl Acad Sci U S A 2015;112(3): 887–92.

26. Erhardt Erik B, Srinivas R, Bedrick Edward J, et al. Comparison of multi-subject ICA methods for analysis of fMRI data. Hum Brain Mapp 2011;32(12): 2075–95.

27. Vesa K, Tapani V, Jukka R, et al. A sliding time-window ICA reveals spatial variability of the default mode network in time. Brain Connect 2011;1(4): 339–47.

28. Airan Raag D, Vogelstein Joshua T, Pillai Jay J, et al. Factors affecting characterization and localization of interindividual differences in functional connectivity using MRI. Hum Brain Mapp 2016;37(5):1986–97.

29. Matthew HR, Thilo W, Allen Elena A, et al. Dynamic functional connectivity: promise, issues, and interpretations. Neuroimage 2013;80:360–78.

30. Johnson Matthew W, Albert G-R, Cosimano Mary P, et al. Pilot study of the 5-HT2AR agonist psilocybin in the treatment of tobacco addiction. J Psychopharmacol 2014;28(11):983–92.

31. Johnson Matthew W, Albert G-R, Griffiths Roland R. Long-term follow-up of psilocybin-facilitated smoking cessation. Am J Drug Alcohol Abuse 2017;43(1):55–60.

32. Ross S, Anthony B, Jeffrey G, et al. Rapid and sustained symptom reduction following psilocybin treatment for anxiety and depression in patients with life-threatening cancer: a randomized controlled trial. J Psychopharmacol 2016;30(12): 1165–80.

33. Carhart-Harris Robin L, Mark B, James R, et al. Psilocybin with psychological support for treatment-resistant depression: an open-label feasibility study. Lancet Psychiatry 2016;3(7):619–27.

34. Enzo T, Robin C-H, Robert L, et al. Enhanced repertoire of brain dynamical states during the psychedelic experience. Hum Brain Mapp 2014;35(11): 5442–56.

35. Madhyastha Tara M, Askren Mary K, Peter B, et al. Dynamic connectivity at rest predicts attention task performance. Brain Connect 2015;5(1):45–59.

36. Aaron K, Arielle T, Sepideh S, et al. Spontaneous cognitive processes and the behavioral validation of time-varying brain connectivity. Netw Neurosci 2018;2(4):397–417.

37. Khambhati Ankit N, Sizemore AE, Betzel Richard F, et al. Modeling and interpreting mesoscale network dynamics. Neuroimage 2018;180:337–49.

38. Murphy AC, Gu S, Khambhati AN, et al. Explicitly Linking Regional Activation and Function Connectivity: Community Structure of Weighted Networks with Continuous Annotation arXiv:1611.07962.

39. Braun U, Axel S, Bassett Danielle S, et al. Dynamic brain network reconfiguration as a potential schizophrenia genetic risk mechanism modulated by NMDA receptor function. Proc Natl Acad Sci U S A 2016;113(44):12568–73.

40. Coyle JT. NMDA receptor and schizophrenia: a brief history. Schizophr Bull 2012;38(5):920–6.

41. Nora L, Van De Ville D. On spurious and real fluctuations of dynamic functional connectivity during rest. Neuroimage 2015;104:430–6.

42. Andrew Z, Breakspear M. Towards a statistical test for functional connectivity dynamics. Neuroimage 2015;114:466–70.

43. Chu Catherine J, Kramer MA, Jay P, et al. Emergence of stable functional networks in long-term human electroencephalography. J Neurosci 2012; 32(8):2703–13.

44. Jones David T, Prashanthi V, Murphy Matthew C, et al. Non-stationarity in the "resting brain's" modular architecture. PLoS One 2012;7(6):e39731.

45. Telesford Qawi K, Mary-Ellen L, Jean V, et al. Detection of functional brain network reconfiguration during task-driven cognitive states. Neuroimage 2016; 142:198–210.

46. Maziar Y, Allen Elena A, Miller Robyn L, et al. Dynamic coherence analysis of resting fMRI data to jointly capture state-based phase, frequency, and time-domain information. Neuroimage 2015;120:133–42.

47. Jia H, Hu X, Gopikrishna D. Behavioral relevance of the dynamics of the functional brain connectome. Brain Connect 2014;4(9):741–59.

48. Waqas M, Matthew M, Wendy H, et al. Spatiotemporal dynamics of low frequency BOLD fluctuations in rats and humans. Neuroimage 2011;54(2): 1140–50.

49. Belloy Michaël E, Maarten N, Anzar A, et al. Dynamic resting state fMRI analysis in mice reveals a set of Quasi-Periodic Patterns and illustrates their relationship with the global signal. Neuroimage 2018;180(Pt B):463–84.

50. Thompson GJ, Pan W-J, Matthew Evan M, et al. Quasi-periodic patterns (QPP): large-scale dynamics in resting state fMRI that correlate with local infraslow electrical activity. Neuroimage 2014;84: 1018–31.

51. Anzar A, Michaël B, Amrit K, et al. Quasi-periodic patterns contribute to functional connectivity in the brain. Neuroimage 2019;191:193–204.

52. Grooms Joshua K, Thompson Garth J, Pan W-J, et al. Infraslow electroencephalographic and dynamic resting state network activity. Brain Connect 2017;7(5):265–80.

53. Lindquist Martin A, Xu Y, Nebel Mary B, et al. Evaluating dynamic bivariate correlations in resting-state fMRI: a comparison study and a new approach. Neuroimage 2014;101:531–46.

54. Sadia S, Chin-Hui L, Keilholz Shella D. Evaluation of sliding window correlation performance for characterizing dynamic functional connectivity and brain states. Neuroimage 2016;133:111–28.

55. Choe Ann S, Nebel Mary B, Barber Anita D, et al. Comparing test-retest reliability of dynamic

functional connectivity methods. Neuroimage 2017; 158:155–75.

56. Roland Jarod L, Hacker Carl D, Snyder Abraham Z, et al. A comparison of resting state functional magnetic resonance imaging to invasive electrocortical stimulation for sensorimotor mapping in pediatric patients. Neuroimage Clin 2019;23:101850.

57. Leuthardt Eric C, Gloria G, Bandt SK, et al. Integration of resting state functional MRI into clinical practice - A large single institution experience. PLoS One 2018;13(6):e0198349.

58. Dierker D, Roland Jarod L, Mudassar K, et al. Resting-state functional magnetic resonance imaging in presurgical functional mapping. Neuroimaging Clin N Am 2017;27(4):621–33.

59. Hacker Carl D, Roland Jarod L, Kim Albert H, et al. Resting-state network mapping in neurosurgical practice: a review. Neurosurg Focus 2019;47(6): E15.

60. O'Connor Erin E, Zeffiro Thomas A. Why is clinical fMRI in a resting state? Front Neurol 2019;10. https://doi.org/10.3389/fneur.2019.00420.

61. Agarwal S, Sair Haris I, Raag A, et al. Demonstration of brain tumor-induced neurovascular uncoupling in resting-state fMRI at ultrahigh field. Brain Connect 2016;6(4):267–72.

62. Chen C, Hou BL, Holodny AI. Effect of Age and Tumor Grade on BOLD fMRI in Preoperative Assessment of Glioma Patients. Radiology 2008;248: 971–8.

63. Abreu VHF, Peck KK, Petrovich-Brennan NM, et al. The influence of tumor pathology and routine MRI Characteristics on BOLD fMRI in the primary motor gyrus in patients with brain tumors. Radiology 2016;281(3):876–83.

64. Sun H, Vachha B, Laino ME, et al. Decreased hand-motor resting-state functional connectivity in patients with glioma: analysis of factors including neurovascular uncoupling. Radiology 2020;294(3): 610–21.

65. Sair Haris I, Yahyavi-Firouz-Abadi N, Calhoun Vince D, et al. Presurgical brain mapping of the language network in patients with brain tumors using resting-state fMRI: comparison with task fMRI. Hum Brain Mapp 2016;37(3):913–23.

66. Yahyavi-Firouz-Abadi N, Pillai JJ, Lindquist MA, et al. Presurgical brain mapping of the ventral somatomotor network in patients with brain tumors using resting-state fMRI. AJNR Am J Neuroradiol 2017; 38(5):1006–12.

67. Wongsripuemtet J, Tyan AE, Carass A, et al. Preoperative mapping of the supplementary motor area in patients with brain tumor using resting-state fMRI with seed-based analysis. Am J Neuroradiol 2018. https://doi.org/10.3174/ajnr.A5709.

68. Syed MF, Lindquist Martin A, Pillai Jay J, et al. Dynamic functional connectivity states between the dorsal and ventral sensorimotor networks revealed by dynamic conditional correlation analysis of resting-state functional magnetic resonance imaging. Brain Connect 2017;7(10):635–42.

Special Articles

Utility of Preoperative Blood-Oxygen-Level–Dependent Functional MR Imaging in Patients with a Central Nervous System Neoplasm

Ammar A. Chaudhry, MD[a],*, Sohaib Naim, BSc[b], Maryam Gul, MD[b],
Abbas Chaudhry, PharmD[b], Mike Chen, MD, PhD[c], Rahul Jandial, MD, PhD[c],
Behnam Badie, MD[c]

KEYWORDS

- fMR imaging brain mapping • BOLD fMR imaging • Sensorimotor • Neurovascular uncoupling

KEY POINTS

- Functional MR imaging provides reliable in vivo assessment of the eloquent cortex and can be used to identify sensorimotor, language, and visual regions.
- Key limitations of BOLD task-fMR imaging include:
  - Necessity of patient cooperation and ability of patients to perform the required task, thus limiting its application in young and elderly patients as well as those with neurocognitive limitations.
  - BOLD fMR imaging is motion sensitive.
  - In instances where tumor involves the eloquent cortex, postoperative changes limit BOLD fMR imaging assessment of perisurgical sites.
  - Tumor and tumor microenvironment can affect normal hemodynamic response, resulting in neurovascular uncoupling and leading to false-negative BOLD fMR imaging signal changes.

INTRODUCTION

Functional neuroimaging provides a means to understand the relationship between brain structure and function.[1] Functional MR (fMR) imaging can offer unique insight into preoperative planning for central nervous system (CNS) neoplasms by identifying areas of the brain affected or spared by the neoplasm.[1] The development of fMR imaging presented a breakthrough in imaging acquisition and analysis[1–3] as well as patient management. Since its discovery in 1992 by Ogawa and colleagues, the blood-oxygen-level–dependent (BOLD) fMR imaging technique has become the dominant in vivo imaging technique for functional brain

This article was previously published in *Radiology Clinics of North America*, Volume 57, Number 6, Pages 1189-1198.

Disclosure Statement: The authors have nothing to disclose.

[a] Precision Imaging Lab, Department of Diagnostic Radiology, City of Hope National Cancer Center, 1500 East Duarte Road, Los Angeles, CA 91010, USA; [b] Department of Diagnostic Radiology, City of Hope National Cancer Center, 1500 East Duarte Road, Los Angeles, CA 91010, USA; [c] Department of Neurosurgery, City of Hope National Cancer Center, 1500 East Duarte Road, Los Angeles, CA 91010, USA

* Corresponding author.

E-mail address: achaudhry@coh.org

Neuroimag Clin N Am 31 (2021) 93–102
https://doi.org/10.1016/j.nic.2020.09.009

imaging. BOLD fMR imaging provides functional information without requiring invasive electrodes, radiation, or intravenous contrast agent.[1,3–5] The BOLD sequence uses differences in tissue magnetic susceptibility properties (T2* effect) between oxyhemoglobin (diamagnetic) and deoxyhemoglobin (paramagnetic).[1,3,4,6] The BOLD fMR imaging signal depends on cerebral blood flow, cerebral blood volume, and cerebral metabolic rate. The net difference between tissue oxyhemoglobin and deoxyhemoglobin during the hemodynamic response (known as the hemodynamic response function [HRF]) is what generates the MR imaging signal. The "BOLD effect" assesses coupling of oxygenated blood flow and neuronal metabolism during functional tasks, resulting in a net difference in oxyhemoglobin and deoxyhemoglobin, which generates the BOLD signal.[3,4,6] Hemoglobin's magnetic properties depend on the reduction-oxidation of iron between Fe^{2+} and Fe^{3+} states (ie, oxygenated and deoxygenated states). These changes result in an increase in local tissue-derived signal intensity on T2*-weighted MR images.[3–7] BOLD fMR imaging provides good spatial resolution for effective mapping of CNS function in patients whose tumor and/or peritumoral edema is adjacent to eloquent cortex.

This article discusses the applications, significance, and interpretation of BOLD fMR imaging and its relevance to presurgical planning in patients with CNS neoplasms.

BLOOD-OXYGEN-LEVEL–DEPENDENT FUNCTIONAL MR IMAGING AND THE ELOQUENT CORTEX
Sensorimotor

At many medical centers in the United States, BOLD fMR imaging is used to evaluate the sensorimotor system by providing an effective, low-risk, noninvasive means of evaluating the eloquent cortex, comparable with intraoperative mapping techniques.[8] BOLD fMR imaging can be used to identify critical areas of interest to the neurosurgeon by discerning key functional areas of gray matter on structural MR imaging. This is particularly important in settings where tumor and/or peritumoral edema is in close proximity to eloquent cortex. The primary motor cortex, located in the precentral gyrus, is responsible for generating neural impulses that control motor movement. Any significant injury to this region can result in irreversible paresis.[1,8,9] The primary sensory cortex is located in the postcentral gyrus.[8] Separated by the central sulcus, the motor and sensory gyri are somatotopically organized.[10]

In the pre-BOLD fMR imaging era and in instances where BOLD fMR imaging is not available, traditional anatomic landmark approaches are used to identify the precentral gyrus and intraoperative electrodes are used to map out the hand-foot motor regions. Traditionally, the "reverse omega sign" is used to identify the hand motor region; however, this is not always reliable to because of anatomic variation and/or distortion of the homunculus by neoplasm or edema. Motor functions activated by the primary somatosensory cortex, such as the planning, execution, and control of specific behavior, is a complex neural process, and delineating neuronal function solely according to anatomic landmarks can be unreliable.[11] In addition, the lack of reliable anatomic landmarks make it difficult to precisely localize the facial motor region on the precentral gyrus.[12] Supported by clinical and neural data, 3 main motor areas (hand, face/lips/tongue, and foot) can be reliably identified on fMR imaging with good agreement between BOLD fMR imaging maps and intraoperative functional mapping.[12,13] The foot motor region is usually located medially along the parasagittal aspect of the precentral gyrus at the level of the interhemispheric fissure (**Figs. 1 and 2**). The direct intraoperative cortical stimulation of this region is complicated by the presence of the adjacent superior sagittal sinus and can be further complicated by the presence of nearby edema, tumor, and/or aberrant vasculature such as a developmental venous anomaly. The 3 main functional areas (face, hand, foot) span the precentral gyrus (lateral to medial) and can be reliably assessed on task-based fMR imaging.[1] It is important that patients with paresis can elicit motor and sensory activation with sensory stimulation of the hand, face, or foot through induced motor signals.[14,15] During an fMR imaging examination, studies have shown paretic patients to induce more head motion as they experience difficulty moving the affected limb, leading to motion artifact and misregistration of BOLD signal.[1]

Also important are secondary motor areas, which when damaged can lead to significant morbidity, thus increasing the importance of precise fMR imaging localization.[1] The secondary areas of the brain of interest for neurosurgical planning include the pre–supplementary motor area (pre-SMA) and the supplementary motor area (SMA).[16] The SMA consists of a posterior SMA, which is most commonly identified adjacent to the precentral sulcus and is normally active during motor tasks (see **Figs. 1 and 2**).[16] The anterior portion of the SMA (**Fig. 3**) is more active during language activation and its borders are less well defined. Recent studies have suggested that the

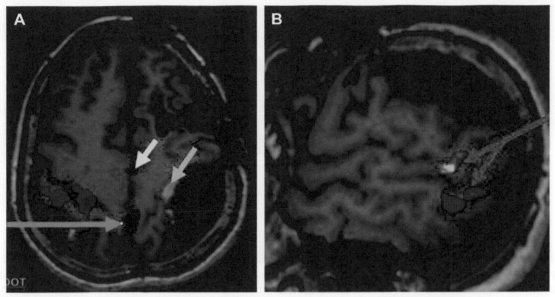

Fig. 1. A 61-year-old woman with recurrent meningioma presented for presurgical evaluation of primary motor cortex. (*A*) Axial T1-precontrast series depicts recurrent extra-axial dural-based mass along the left posterior cerebral convexity with mass effect on the perirolandic structures. Task-fMR imaging BOLD signal depicts motor activation along the precentral gyrus (left foot, *green arrow*; left hand, *orange arrow*; SMA, *yellow arrow*). (*B*) Sagittal T1-precontrast images in the same subject depicts Wernicke area (*blue arrows*) along the posterolateral left temporal lobe with variant anatomy.

motor region of the SMA is somatotopically arranged.[16] Studies have shown that direct activation of the SMA influences speech, which is evident during different language tasks, such as

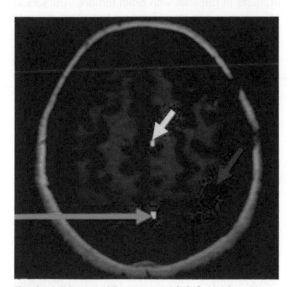

Fig. 2. A 36-year-old woman with left insular glioma presented for preoperative eloquent cortex mapping. Left toe movement elicits activation in the left parasagittal precentral gyrus (*green arrow*), and left finger tap elicits activation along the lateral aspect of the left precentral gyrus (*red arrow*). The SMA is depicted by the yellow arrow.

silent verbal fluency and repetition.[17] Motor planning is largely associated with the SMA. Within the SMA is a centralized region that remains active during both language and motor tasks. It is also acknowledged that the SMA plays an important role in the planning and execution of movements, and that both passive and active tasks can be reliably detected through BOLD fMR imaging.[17]

Because surgical resection of a brain neoplasm poses a risk to the eloquent cortex with potential for permanent neurologic damage, preoperative BOLD fMR imaging is particularly useful in cases where tumor and/or peritumoral edema is in close proximity to eloquent cortex. Using fMR imaging techniques, surgical teams can plan tumor resection through noninvasive visualization of the brain and analysis of lesion localization in relation to anatomic landmarks.[18] Furthermore, fMR imaging derived information can also be used in counseling patients about the risks involved with surgical resection and in prospectively developing an appropriate surgical approach.[19]

Language (Broca and Wernicke Areas) and Memory

The Intracarotid Amobarbital Test, otherwise known as "Wada" testing, has been considered the gold standard for determining the language-dominant hemisphere.[20] Although it is well known

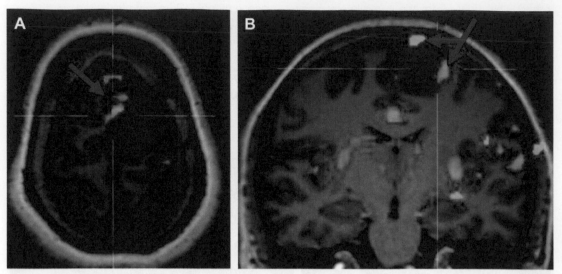

Fig. 3. Axial (*A*) and coronal (*B*) presurgical task-fMR imaging in a 39-year-old woman with history of left frontal oligodendroglioma depicts SMA (*red arrow*) along the anteromedial and lateral margins of the neoplasm, which was confirmed on intraoperative functional mapping.

that the left cerebral hemisphere is usually the dominant center for language in most of the population, adequate preoperative testing is required to properly establish cerebral language dominance (**Fig. 4**). Owing to its high level of accuracy in predicting hemispheric language dominance and its noninvasive nature, task-fMR imaging is the standard of care in medical centers where it is available. Silent word-generation paradigms are most commonly used to elicit activation in the Broca area, most commonly located in the inferior frontal gyrus (**Fig. 5**). Silent sentence completion is the most frequently used paradigm to elicit activation in the Wernicke area (see **Fig. 5**). Of importance is that language regions (Wernicke more so than Broca) tend to be somewhat more broadly distributed and require careful image acquisition and postprocessing to ensure accurate depiction of the language network and limit overestimation or underestimation of these regions. To improve precision of localizing Broca and Wernicke regional activity, additional language paradigms are delivered including rhyming, antonym generation, object naming, and/or passive story listening.

Evaluation of memory lateralization is not well established on task-fMR imaging. A case study by Szaflarski and colleagues[21] showed mixed results in the diagnostic accuracy of fMR imaging in predicting the memory outcomes of patients with epilepsy through presurgical evaluation. At present, additional research is required to develop a robust task-fMR or resting state fMR (rs-fMR) imaging application for memory assessment. Such a development can be applied in the

preoperative setting for patients with tumor or epilepsy, but can also be extended to evaluation of neurodegenerative diseases.[10]

PITFALLS OF BLOOD-OXYGEN-LEVEL–DEPENDENT FUNCTIONAL MR IMAGING

During an fMR imaging scan, it is common to find artifacts in patients with brain tumors. Artifacts in MR imaging can result from anything that disrupts the T2* imaging signal, and may be caused by the MR scanner hardware or patient interaction.[22]

Motion-related artifacts can be random or episodic (essential tremor, breathing, cardiac related) and are usually minor in amplitude. As such, most fMR imaging postprocessing software packages are robust enough to remove noise and adequately coregister BOLD and structural MR imaging series. Stimulus-related motion (eg, facial movement during word generation or sentence rhyming) can be difficult to remove. With modern statistical analysis, these motion-related signal artifacts may be removed as long as they vary enough from signal generated by the stimulus presentation. It is noteworthy that significant motion artifact can limit the BOLD series' diagnostic value and can be difficult to remove with standard motion correction. This artifact can affect stimulus-related BOLD signal and structural correlation, and be mistaken for the stimulus-generated signal, adversely affecting the study.[1] A strategy to overcome this limitation is to use the contralateral hemisphere as a reference control to simplify suppositions about displaced anatomy and affected

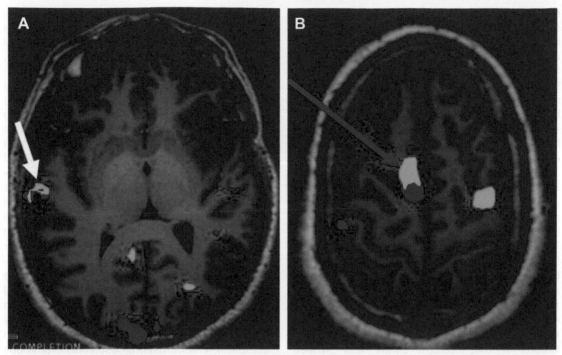

Fig. 4. Preoperative axial task-fMR imaging (*A*) in a 29-year-old man with left frontoinsular glioma depicts right temporal dominance of Wernicke area (*white arrow*). More superiorly, (*B*) there is robust activation of the SMA in the right frontal lobe (*red arrow*).

BOLD signal magnitudes.[23] In such cases, repeat acquisition is recommended.

The BOLD fMR imaging signal can be attenuated by noise. Multi-echo echo-planar (EP)

imaging, whereby the fMR imaging signal is collected at multiple echo times, is a method to improve sensitivity to BOLD responses.[24] This allows for better noise reduction capability and

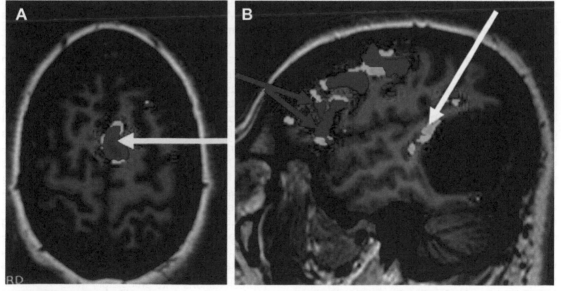

Fig. 5. Preoperative axial task-fMR imaging (*A*) in a 31-year-old man with left temporo-occipital glioma depicts left cerebral language dominance with robust activation of the SMA in the left frontal lobe (*yellow arrow*). Sagittal series (*B*) depicts activation in Broca (*red arrow*) and Wernicke (*white arrow*) regions.

offers advantages in imaging brain regions susceptible to distortion and signal dropout.[24] It is important to routinely inspect T2*-weighted images in an attempt to correct any and all artifacts found during the fMR imaging scans. As BOLD fMR imaging is an EP imaging–based technique, susceptibility artifact can result in BOLD signal loss, for example in blood products (hemosiderin), air-tissue interface, and metal (eg, dental hardware, surgical hardware near cortical regions).[1]

Neurovascular uncoupling (NVU), which refers to disruption of coupling between neuronal activity and neurovascular response in areas within or surrounding the tumor, is a major pitfall to consider, as it can lead to false-negative neuronal activity. The BOLD effect is proportional to the net change in volume from oxygenated to deoxygenated blood in the tissue; this is true as long as the natural HRF between the neurovascular system and the brain is preserved. In certain conditions—for example, hypervascular neoplasms—the normal HRF is disrupted, predisposing to NVU. As such, lesions in the eloquent cortex with marked increased vascularity should be scrutinized closely in cases demonstrating limited to no significant neuronal activation.[1]

BLOOD-OXYGEN-LEVEL–DEPENDENT FUNCTIONAL MR IMAGING APPLICATIONS

BOLD fMR imaging can reliably map eloquent cortex presurgically and is sufficiently accurate for neurosurgical planning. HRF captured on BOLD fMR imaging allows for noninvasive in vivo assessment of eloquent cortical activation.[25] BOLD fMR imaging is useful for identification of the primary sensorimotor cortex, especially in cases where gyral anatomy is distorted by neoplasm or other CNS disorder (see **Fig. 1**). In patients with brain tumors undergoing neurosurgical intervention, fMR imaging can decrease postoperative morbidity by identifying eloquent cortex prospectively to guide surgical intervention. BOLD fMR imaging can be performed to evaluate the sensorimotor regions with paradigms that are both volitional and passive.[26] Normal brain anatomic variance (see **Fig. 1**) is another reason patients undergo fMR imaging, because the conventional anatomic landmarks associated with functional brain regions cannot be identified on structural imaging.[26,27]

Neuroplasticity refers to the reorganization of neural networks that can be seen in the setting of slow-growing neoplasms and is another key factor to be considered in functional recovery of patients with brain tumors. fMR imaging can help identify reorganization in cerebral networks prospectively, guiding appropriate surgical intervention and minimizing postoperative morbidity.[28] In patients with CNS neoplasms and history of stroke or comorbidities (eg, hypertension, coronary artery disease, diabetes) placing them at risk for stroke, fMR imaging can help depict reorganization of functional networks. Studies have shown that performing simple motor tasks with the affected limb following a stroke is associated with higher brain activation in many cortical areas when compared with healthy volunteers, including regions of the dorsal motor cortex, the ventral motor cortex, and the SMA.[28] Longitudinal fMR imaging studies have revealed that neural activity is often enhanced in motion-related areas in both hemispheres before returning to normal levels similar to those in healthy controls during the first 12 months after stroke.[3]

Numerous other considerations are important when performing BOLD fMR imaging in clinical practice. For example, patients with brain tumors benefit from shorter-length tasks because they find greater difficulty keeping their head still in comparison with healthy subjects. Numerous studies have shown that patients benefit from signal averaging via block design, meaning that brain regions associated with a specific task can be activated even if it is not essential to the task being performed.[29] For example, since the primary visual cortex shows robust activation on language fMR imaging paradigms, the authors reduce the overall scan time in patients in whom the visual cortex is uninvolved by acquiring information of the primary visual cortex on language paradigms and excluding visual paradigms from the fMR imaging examinations. The authors perform fMR imaging examinations with dedicated visual paradigms in cases where the patient is symptomatic (visual deficits), or when the primary visual cortical region is infiltrated by neoplasm or distorted by mass effect. Similarly, in instances when eloquent cortex is distant from pathology and functional deficits are not clinically detected, fMR imaging examinations are curtailed to reduce scan time for patient comfort. This strategy is also helpful in instances where the patient is projected to undergo a longer than usual MR imaging evaluation (eg, MR imaging spectroscopy).

BOLD fMR imaging in the postoperative setting is especially helpful if a patient is expected to undergo staged and/or multistep surgical resection. For example, after a tumor is removed, regions of brain compressed by mass effect may demonstrate regained functionality because this tissue can become active, showing the BOLD effect on postoperative fMR imaging.

TASK-BASED VERSUS RESTING-STATE BLOOD-OXYGEN-LEVEL–DEPENDENT FUNCTIONAL MR IMAGING

To elicit neuronal activation for generation of BOLD signal, patients are trained before entering the MR imaging scanner and instructed to follow tasks delivered in functional paradigms given as visual cues. For motor cortex activation (see Fig. 2), foot movement, finger tapping, and lip pucker (or tongue movement) are most commonly used. For language network assessment (Fig. 6), silent word generation, sentence completion, and rhyming are the 3 most commonly used paradigms. To limit scan variability, the American Society of Functional Neuroradiology has provided a list of paradigms with recommended scanner parameters (https://www.asfnr.org/paradigms/).

Task-fMR imaging depends on the patient's ability to perform specific tasks that elicit BOLD signal alternation on MR imaging. The BOLD series is overlaid on the structural imaging (usually high-resolution T1 and/or T2-weighted sequence) to locate eloquent regions such as the primary language and motor and visual cortices.[1–3] There are several Food and Drug Administration–approved commercial software packages available in clinical practice that have made evaluation of task-based fMR imaging less time consuming by automating most of the postprocessing (eg, motion correction, image registration).

Though reliable in most clinical settings, task-based fMR imaging presents certain limitations and disadvantages. For example, task-based fMR imaging cannot be performed in patients suffering from severe neurologic deficits (eg, dementia, complete paresis).[30] Depending on language limitations and/or educational barriers, several different tasks may be required to assess different motor and language functions. Many trials may be required to achieve the desired activation maps, resulting in lengthy scanning sessions.[30] Task-fMR imaging also has limited utility in the pediatric preadolescent setting (especially infants and toddlers) because of the required cooperation by patients, as these subjects cannot follow commands on task-paradigms that are usually delivered through visual cues.

rs-fMR imaging is another BOLD fMR imaging technique with potential for overcoming task-based limitations. rs-fMR imaging measures the BOLD effect over a period of time while the patient is in the MR scanner. Agarwal and colleagues[31] had originally measured the resting state of the human brain motor cortex with fMR imaging and discovered that even during rest, different brain regions are able to communicate without an actively performed task. Because there are no prescan training requirements of the subject for rs-fMR imaging scanning, patients can be instructed to lie quietly with their eyes closed during the scanning process.[31] rs-fMR imaging is emerging as a useful alternative to task-fMR imaging, especially in cases where task-fMR imaging cannot be performed. In the absence of task performance, rs-fMR imaging maps acquire BOLD signal corresponding to low-frequency neuronal signal fluctuations during rest, thus allowing for detection of multiple functional networks.[31] By using the changes in the BOLD signal, a 4-dimensional time series of the brain can be constructed to reflect changing neuronal activity.[6] As the data are processed through a series of steps including

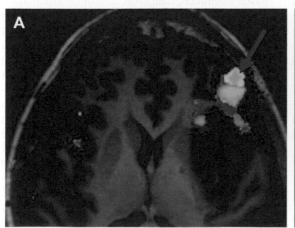
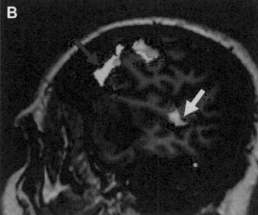

Fig. 6. A 42-year-old man with left insular glioma presented for presurgical language network mapping. fMR imaging depicts left cerebral dominance of the language network with robust activation in (A) Broca region (red arrow) and (B) Wernicke region (yellow arrow).

head motion correction, spatial smoothing, and noise and bandpass filtering, the data can be evaluated.[6] Multiple subject comparison requires normalization of the data across all subjects followed by a method of targeting the connection between the regions.

The most popular analysis methods for targeting connections include seed-based analysis (SBA) and independent component analysis (ICA). SBA is a hypothesis-driven method that uses an extracted BOLD time course from the region of interest (ROI) to determine the connectivity of a seed relative to the rest of the brain.[32] ICA is a mathematical technique used to define a region of functional connectivity. ICA is a data-driven technique used to decompose the data set into independent components with strong temporal coherence (intraconnected maps), each of which associates with the time course of the overall signal.[4,32] Although the application of fMR imaging in neuro-oncology has become standard in localizing brain regions before surgery, there has been difficulty in transitioning from task-based localization to the resting state.

A key limitation in rs-fMR imaging has been the lack of standardization across many recent studies. Although new fMR imaging technologies are being developed, there is a lack of standardization of physiologic parameters, pharmacologic interventions, and characterization of disease-related vascular changes, with limited concrete data on how these changes affect the BOLD signal.[33] Current methods to analyze data also have limitations. SBA is based on predetermined ROIs, which can be arbitrary or task-fMR imaging derived.[24] Because some patients may have brain-distorting mass lesions, the collective database of ROIs may become difficult to use.[6,24] Although the uses of task versus rs-fMR imaging techniques differ in reliability to functional mapping, certain approaches see similar reliability with respect to mapping the sensorimotor network of healthy subjects. rs-fMR imaging has shown great promise as a diagnostic tool, and with enough comparative studies showing lack of discrepancy between both task and rs-fMR imaging, it has potential to become the noninvasive standard of care for surgical planning and prognosis.[30–33]

COMBINATION FUNCTIONAL BRAIN IMAGING

For presurgical planning, many techniques can be implemented complementarily to fMR imaging. Techniques used in place of or in addition to fMR imaging are magnetoencephalography (MEG), electroencephalography (EEG), PET, and diffusion tractography (DTI).[1] Different techniques can vary in spatial or temporal resolution, invasiveness, and how they localize or lateralize function.

MEG has been shown to predict the location of the gyrus of interest more accurately and specifically in comparison with fMR imaging.[34] Because fMR imaging activates the entire network (both primary and secondary areas) for motor tasks, there is difficulty interpreting where the primary, secondary, and sensory gyri are localized because they are acting simultaneously. This is not an issue with MEG. Spatial resolution between the 2 methods vary such that fMR imaging can be as low as 1 mm, whereas MEG achieves 5 mm.[34–36] Both techniques assist in more precise preoperative surgical planning compared with traditional MR markers, however, because MEG scanners are not as readily available as conventional MR imaging scanners, the latter being more commonly used.[1]

EEG is a method similar to MEG in that it directly measures electrical activity of the brain through small metal electrodes.[34] Even though intraoperative EEG is traditionally more invasive than fMR imaging, integrating the 2 techniques into the neurosurgical navigation system is beneficial in certain cases.

DTI is an MR technique that measures water diffusivity along white matter tracts using eigenvectors.[2,3] In particular, DTI is able to map and characterize diffusion as a function of spatial localization.[2,3] The combination of DTI with other imaging methods can improve its specificity for complex diseases. Combining DTI with gray matter fMR imaging localization paints a more complete picture of the functional anatomy in the area surrounding a tumor, with feedback such as tissue infiltration, distortion, and/or destruction.[1–3]

PET imaging can provide functional information by using a radioactive imaging agent conjugated with another compound (eg, glucose, antibodies, small molecules) depending on the disease of interest.[20,37] Fluorodeoxyglucose (FDG), a glucose analog, is the most commonly used PET radiotracer that provides metabolic information associated with tumor. FDG PET's role is somewhat limited in the setting of CNS neoplasms because there is increased background brain parenchymal FDG uptake resulting from physiologic neuronal activity, which limits spatial discrimination between tumor and adjacent normal brain tissue.[38] PET-MR imaging is a hybrid technology allowing for simultaneous acquisition of both PET and MR.[39] The benefit of the PET-MR imaging is that it can provide improved spatial resolution of detected CNS abnormalities with less (about

50%) PET radiotracer-associated radiation exposure.[39] In CNS disorders, PET-MR imaging scans are most commonly used for evaluation of neoplasms, epilepsy, and neurodegenerative disorders.

SUMMARY

Functional neuroimaging is integral to current clinical practice in various disciplines including neuro-oncology, neurodegenerative disorders, and epilepsy. BOLD fMR imaging has been shown to help in presurgical planning, minimizing the risk of postsurgical morbidity while reducing operative time and decreasing craniotomy size.[3,6] Task-based BOLD fMR imaging is the most commonly used technique for noninvasive assessment of eloquent cortex[2,3,6] and can reliably elucidate cortical regions involved in sensorimotor, language, and visual functions. Though reliable, it is important to be aware of pitfalls of this technique, such as neurovascular uncoupling and susceptibility artifact, so as to provide the most accurate functional assessment.

ACKNOWLEDGMENTS

Funding support: Dr A.A. Chaudhry received funding support from NIH 5K12CA001727-23 and City of Hope Young Investigator Award. The authors would like to acknowledge Seth Hilliard for his assistance with the literature search on this article.

REFERENCES

1. Gabriel M, Brennan NP, Peck KK, et al. Blood oxygen level dependent functional magnetic resonance imaging for presurgical planning. Neuroimaging Clin N Am 2014;24(4):557–71.
2. Ulmer JL, Klein AP, Mueller WM, et al. Preoperative diffusion tensor imaging: improving neurosurgical outcomes in brain tumor patients. Neuroimaging Clin N Am 2014;24(4):599–617.
3. Filippi M, Agosta F. Diffusion tensor imaging and functional MRI. Handb Clin Neurol 2016;136: 1065–87.
4. Yeh CJ, Tseng YS, Lin YR, et al. Resting-state functional magnetic resonance imaging: the impact of regression analysis. J Neuroimaging 2015;25(1): 117–23.
5. Buchbinder BR. Functional magnetic resonance imaging. Handb Clin Neurol 2016;135:61–92.
6. Lang S, Duncan N, Northoff G. Resting-state functional magnetic resonance imaging: review of neurosurgical applications. Neurosurgery 2014;74(5): 453–64 [discussion: 464–5].
7. Dimou S, Battisti RA, Hermens DF, et al. A systematic review of functional magnetic resonance imaging and diffusion tensor imaging modalities used in presurgical planning of brain tumour resection. Neurosurg Rev 2013;36(2): 205–14 [discussion: 214].
8. Buxton RB. The physics of functional magnetic resonance imaging (fMRI). Rep Prog Phys 2013;76(9): 096601.
9. Mangraviti A, Casali C, Cordella R, et al. Practical assessment of preoperative functional mapping techniques: navigated transcranial magnetic stimulation and functional magnetic resonance imaging. Neurol Sci 2013;34(9):1551–7.
10. Barras CD, Asadi H, Baldeweg T, et al. Functional magnetic resonance imaging in clinical practice: state of the art and science. Aust Fam Physician 2016;45(11):798–803.
11. Borich MR, Brodie SM, Gray WA, et al. Understanding the role of the primary somatosensory cortex: opportunities for rehabilitation. Neuropsychologia 2015;79(Pt B):246–55.
12. Silva MA, See AP, Essayed WI, et al. Challenges and techniques for presurgical brain mapping with functional MRI. Neuroimage Clin 2018;17: 794–803.
13. Leisman G, Moustafa AA, Shafir T. Thinking, walking, talking: integratory motor and cognitive brain function. Front Public Health 2016;4:94.
14. Reid LB, Boyd RN, Cunnington R, et al. Interpreting intervention induced neuroplasticity with fMRI: the case for multimodal imaging strategies. Neural Plast 2016;2016:2643491.
15. Hassa T, de Jel E, Tuescher O, et al. Functional networks of motor inhibition in conversion disorder patients and feigning subjects. Neuroimage Clin 2016;11:719–27.
16. Potgieser AR, de Jong BM, Wagemakers M, et al. Insights from the supplementary motor area syndrome in balancing movement initiation and inhibition. Front Hum Neurosci 2014;8:960.
17. Vergani F, Lacerda L, Martino J, et al. White matter connections of the supplementary motor area in humans. J Neurol Neurosurg Psychiatry 2014;85(12): 1377–85.
18. Yu ZB, Lv YB, Song LH, et al. Functional connectivity differences in the insular sub-regions in migraine without aura: a resting-state functional magnetic resonance imaging study. Front Behav Neurosci 2017;11:124.
19. Abalkhail TM, MacDonald DB, Al Thubaiti I, et al. Intraoperative direct cortical stimulation motor evoked potentials: stimulus parameter recommendations based on rheobase and chronaxie. Clin Neurophysiol 2017;128(11):2300–8.
20. Benjamin CFA, Dhingra I, Li AX, et al. Presurgical language fMRI: technical practices in epilepsy surgical planning. Hum Brain Mapp 2018;39(10): 4032–42.

21. Szaflarski JP, Gloss D, Binder JR, et al. Practice guideline summary: use of fMRI in the presurgical evaluation of patients with epilepsy: report of the guideline development, dissemination, and implementation Subcommittee of the American Academy of Neurology. Neurology 2017;88(4):395–402.

22. Krupa K, Bekiesinska-Figatowska M. Artifacts in magnetic resonance imaging. Pol J Radiol 2015; 80:93–106.

23. Middlebrooks EH, Frost CJ, Tuna IS, et al. Reduction of motion artifacts and noise using independent component analysis in task-based functional MRI for preoperative planning in patients with brain tumor. AJNR Am J Neuroradiol 2017;38(2):336–42.

24. Caballero-Gaudes C, Reynolds RC. Methods for cleaning the BOLD fMRI signal. Neuroimage 2017; 154:128–49.

25. Dewiputri WI, Auer T. Functional magnetic resonance imaging (FMRI) neurofeedback: implementations and applications. Malays J Med Sci 2013; 20(5):5–15.

26. Choudhri AF, Patel RM, Siddiqui A, et al. Cortical activation through passive-motion functional MRI. AJNR Am J Neuroradiol 2015;36(9):1675–81.

27. Durning SJ, Costanzo M, Artino AR Jr, et al. Using functional magnetic resonance imaging to improve how we understand, teach, and assess clinical reasoning. J Contin Educ Health Prof 2014;34(1): 76–82.

28. Li W, Wang M, Li Y, et al. A novel brain network construction method for exploring age-related functional reorganization. Comput Intell Neurosci 2016;2016: 2429691.

29. Abd-El-Barr MM, Saleh E, Huang RY, et al. Effect of disease and recovery on functional anatomy in brain tumor patients: insights from functional MRI and diffusion tensor imaging. Imaging Med 2013;5(4): 333–46.

30. Palacios EM, Sala-Llonch R, Junque C, et al. Resting-state functional magnetic resonance imaging activity and connectivity and cognitive outcome in traumatic brain injury. JAMA Neurol 2013;70(7): 845–51.

31. Agarwal S, Lu H, Pillai JJ. Value of frequency domain resting-state functional magnetic resonance imaging metrics amplitude of low-frequency fluctuation and fractional amplitude of low-frequency fluctuation in the assessment of brain tumor-induced neurovascular uncoupling. Brain Connect 2017;7(6):382–9.

32. Wu L, Caprihan A, Bustillo J, et al. An approach to directly link ICA and seed-based functional connectivity: application to schizophrenia. Neuroimage 2018;179:448–70.

33. Chen JE, Glover GH. Functional magnetic resonance imaging methods. Neuropsychol Rev 2015; 25(3):289–313.

34. Proudfoot M, Woolrich MW, Nobre AC, et al. Magnetoencephalography. Pract Neurol 2014;14(5): 336–43.

35. Schmid E, Thomschewski A, Taylor A, et al, E-PILEPSY consortium. Diagnostic accuracy of functional magnetic resonance imaging, Wada test, magnetoencephalography, and functional transcranial Doppler sonography for memory and language outcome after epilepsy surgery: a systematic review. Epilepsia 2018. https://doi.org/10.1111/epi.14588.

36. Sollmann N, Ille S, Boeckh-Behrens T, et al. Mapping of cortical language function by functional magnetic resonance imaging and repetitive navigated transcranial magnetic stimulation in 40 healthy subjects. Acta Neurochir (Wien) 2016;158(7):1303–16.

37. Bruinsma TJ, Sarma VV, Oh Y, et al. The relationship between dopamine neurotransmitter dynamics and the blood-oxygen-level-dependent (BOLD) Signal: a review of pharmacological functional magnetic resonance imaging. Front Neurosci 2018;12:238.

38. Smucny J, Wylie KP, Tregellas JR. Functional magnetic resonance imaging of intrinsic brain networks for translational drug discovery. Trends Pharmacol Sci 2014;35(8):397–403.

39. Matthews R, Choi M. Clinical utility of positron emission tomography magnetic resonance imaging (PET-MRI) in gastrointestinal cancers. Diagnostics (Basel) 2016;6(3). https://doi.org/10.3390/diagnostics 6030035.

Imaging Glioblastoma Posttreatment
Progression, Pseudoprogression, Pseudoresponse, Radiation Necrosis

Sara B. Strauss, MD, Alicia Meng, MD, Edward J. Ebani, MD, Gloria C. Chiang, MD*

KEYWORDS

- Glioblastoma • Pseudoprogression • Pseudoresponse • Radiation necrosis

KEY POINTS

- Various assessment guidelines for tumor progression, primarily designed for the purpose of phase 2 clinical trials, have been used over the course of the past several decades, with changes over time reflecting evolution in the approach to treatment and technological advances in imaging.
- Radiation necrosis and pseudoprogression are often thought of as 2 opposite extremes on the spectrum of radiation-induced injury, and imaging features may mimic disease progression.
- Pseudoresponse occurs in the setting of antiangiogenic therapy, and imaging findings include decreased contrast enhancement, edema, and permeability as early as 1 day after initiation of therapy.
- A multimodality approach to treatment response coupled with an understanding of the strengths and limitations of various imaging techniques is essential to accurate assessment of treatment response.

INTRODUCTION

Eighty percent of all malignant primary brain tumors diagnosed in the United States are gliomas.[1] The current treatment paradigm for high-grade gliomas (grades III and IV) includes maximal surgical resection followed by concurrent adjuvant radiation and chemotherapy. The relatively recent addition of adjuvant chemotherapy with an oral alkylating agent, temozolomide, is based on pivotal data published in 2005 by Stupp and colleagues,[2] which demonstrated a clinically meaningful and statistically significant overall survival benefit with minimal additional toxicity.

For patients with primary treatment failure or recurrence, the Food and Drug Administration approved the use of bevacizumab, an anti–vascular endothelial growth factor (VEGF) monoclonal antibody, in 2009.[3] In addition, there are many experimental therapies currently under active investigation for patients with recurrent glioblastoma. These include immunomodulatory approaches, such as immune checkpoint inhibitors, tumor vaccines, chimeric antigen receptor (CAR)-modified T-cell therapy, and oncolytic virotherapy. Recently developed immune checkpoint inhibitors such as anti-CTLA-4 (ipilimumab) and anti-PD-1 (pembrolizumab and nivolumab) antibodies have demonstrated clinical efficacy in several solid tumors, with clinical trials for glioblastoma ongoing. Examples of viruses currently under investigation in patients with recurrent glioblastoma include an

This article was previously published in *Radiology Clinics of North America*, Volume 57, Number 6, Pages 1199-1216.

Disclosure Statement: The authors have no conflicts of interest to disclose.

Department of Radiology, Weill Cornell Medical Center, 525 East 68th Street, Box 141, New York, NY 10065, USA

* Corresponding author.

E-mail address: gcc9004@med.cornell.edu

adenovirus expressing interleukin (IL)-12, a herpes simplex virus–1 replicating strain expressing IL-12, vaccine strains of the measles virus, an attenuated poliovirus vaccine, and a replicating retrovirus. Finally, alternating electric field therapy in which a portable device is attached to the scalp and delivers continuous low-intensity alternating electric fields has demonstrated prolonged progression-free and overall survival when used in combination with standard therapy. The device was approved in 2015 for the treatment of newly diagnosed glioblastoma and is expected to change the standard of care.[4]

Tumor recurrence occurs in patients within a median of 6.7 months,[5] with mean overall survival time of 14 to 16 months for glioblastomas.[2,6] Radiographic monitoring of response is key, with a recent publication proposing a standardized reporting template for posttreatment glioma, including tumor genetics (isocitrate dehydrogenase [IDH], O^6-methylguanine-DNA methyltransferase [MGMT] promoter) and treatment history.[7] The purpose of this review was to detail the imaging appearance of 4 key diagnoses in posttreatment glioma surveillance: true progression, pseudoprogression, pseudoresponse, and radiation necrosis.

CONVENTIONAL IMAGING: EVOLUTION OF ASSESSMENT CRITERIA
Progression

Various assessment guidelines for tumor progression, primarily designed for the purpose of phase 2 clinical trials, have been used over the course of the past several decades. Changes over time reflect evolution in the approach to treatment and technological advances in imaging.

The Levin criteria was a numerical grading system introduced in 1977, and imaging features important to diagnosis included size of tumor, central lucency, degree of contrast enhancement, surrounding edema, and ventricle size.[8] In 1990, the Macdonald criteria were published, relying heavily on maximal cross-sectional tumor measurements; these became the most widely used assessment guidelines for the ensuing 20 years.[9,10] The 2-dimensional approach to lesion measurement of the Macdonald criteria was replaced with the application of unidimensional measurement in the Response Evaluation Criteria in Solid Tumors (RECIST) guidelines to gliomas, defining progression by at least a 20% increase in the sum of the diameters of all target lesions, with a maximum of 5 lesions targeted for measurement.[11]

In 2010, the RANO (Response Assessment in Neurooncology) guidelines were introduced, and progression was defined based on imaging features as well as time from completion of chemoradiation (<12 weeks and >12 weeks); important factors in determining progression included enhancement outside of the radiation field, increase by 25% or greater in the sum of the products of perpendicular diameters between the first post-radiotherapy (RT) scan and the scan 12 weeks later, or clinical deterioration. The RANO guidelines additionally consider use of anti-angiogenics; increase in T2/fluid-attenuated inversion recovery (FLAIR) signal in nonenhancing lesions in such patients is indicative of disease progression.[12] With the increased use of immunotherapy, the RANO in immunotherapy guidelines were introduced, which defined imaging criteria less than 6 months and more than 6 months after start of immunotherapy,[13] given that there may be a latency period during which disease may actually worsen while the effective immune response evolves.[14] Importantly, increase or decrease in steroid dose within 2 weeks of MR imaging assessment make disease progression non-evaluable according to the iRANO criteria.[13] The modified RANO criteria were published in 2017 with increased focus on pseudoprogression, and with progressive disease determination based on at least 2 sequential studies, separated by 4 weeks, showing 25% or more increase in size; any new measurable lesion requires confirmation on a repeat study 4 weeks later, clear clinical deterioration, or lack of repeat evaluation due to deteriorating condition/death.[15] The RANO criteria and subsequent modifications highlight the quandary behind many posttreatment glioma cases: both true disease progression and pseudoprogression can present with increased tumor enhancement. In fact, new enhancement seen within the radiation field within the first 12 weeks after treatment can never be definitively diagnosed as progression versus pseudoprogression based on the RANO guidelines.

The following sections cover both conventional and advanced imaging approaches to differentiating between these various entities.

DEFINITION OF PSEUDOPROGRESSION

Pseudoprogression is defined as radiographic evidence of disease progression, typically within 3 to 6 months posttreatment, followed by spontaneous resolution or improvement without additional treatment.[16,17] Pseudoprogression may be accompanied by symptoms in 21% to 34% of patients with high-grade gliomas, but may be asymptomatic in patients with low-grade gliomas, particularly in the adult population.[18] The pathophysiology of pseudoprogression is distinct from radiation necrosis, and likely relates to endothelial cell injury resulting in tissue inflammation and upregulation of VEGF leading to increased vessel permeability and edema, an effect potentiated by chemotherapy administration.[16] In addition to high-grade gliomas, low-grade (World Health Organization [WHO] II) gliomas and WHO III (IDH mutant) gliomas also can demonstrate pseudoprogression.[19–21] Studies have shown that ultimately, patients with pseudoprogression have better outcomes,[20,22] presumably because pseudoprogression reflects an augmented response to treatment.

Early recognition of the concept of pseudoprogression in the setting of radiotherapy led to the suggestion that patients with radiological evidence of progressive disease within the first 3 months of treatment be excluded from phase 2 trials.[23] It was subsequently learned that concurrent treatment with RT and chemotherapy potentiated the effects of radiation necrosis,[24] leading to earlier manifestation of pseudoprogression after treatment initiation. Misinterpretation of pseudoprogression is problematic in terms of patient assignment to clinical trials, interpretation of trial results, guidance of decisions regarding reoperation, and in contributing to patient anxiety.[25] Prospective identification of pseudoprogression can be radiologically and even histologically challenging,[26] and inconsistency in the definition of pseudoprogression confounds comparison between studies. **Figs. 1** and **2** illustrate examples of biopsy-proven progression and pseudoprogression, respectively.

FACTORS ASSOCIATED WITH PSEUDOPROGRESSION

Factors associated with pseudoprogression include cancer genotype and radiation dose. MGMT methylation is associated with increased probability of pseudoprogression and better outcomes.[27–29] For instance, in a group of 157 patients with glioblastoma multiforme, IDH1 mutation, and MGMT methylation predicted a high probability of pseudoprogression, as well as improved overall survival.[30] The incidence of pseudoprogression in patients with MGMT methylated tumor genetics was shown to be 91% compared with 41% in patients with the unmethylated promotor.[31] IDH1 mutation was shown to have high specificity in the detection of pseudoprogression in a study of 32 patients with GBM treated with temozolomide and radiotherapy.[32] Dose of radiotherapy also impacts likelihood of pseudoprogression[2,16] and among patients with lower-grade glioma, proton therapy results in higher prevalence

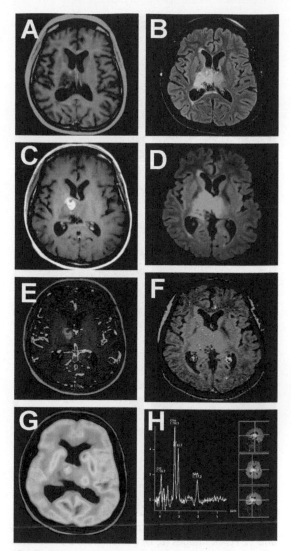

Fig. 1. True progression. Axial postcontrast 3-dimensional T1 SPACE (*A, C*) and T2 FLAIR images (*B, D*) demonstrating a bithalamic infiltrative anaplastic astrocytoma (*B*) with a small enhancing nodule in the right anterior thalamus (*A*). A month later, the enhancing nodule increased significantly in size (*C*), with increased T2 hyperintensity and local mass effect (*D*). DCE-MR perfusion was performed to help evaluate the degree of tumor angiogenesis. Region-of-interest interrogation of the enhancing nodule on the Vp map, superimposed on the postcontrast T1 (*E*), demonstrated markedly elevated plasma volume relative to contralateral thalamus and normal-appearing white matter. As evident on the Ktrans map, superimposed on the T2 FLAIR (*F*), there was also associated elevated permeability. An image from the integrated PET-MR study demonstrated elevated FDG uptake in the enhancing nodule (*G*). Single-voxel MRS (*H*) demonstrated an elevated choline-to-NAA ratio, also compatible with tumor metabolism. Subsequent surgical biopsy confirmed tumor progression.

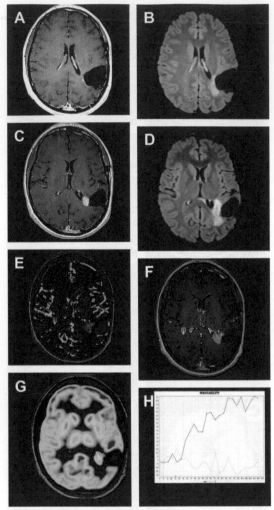

Fig. 2. Pseudoprogression. Axial postcontrast T1 (*A, C*) and T2 FLAIR images (*B, D*) demonstrate a small focus of enhancement along the medial margin of the resection cavity (*A*) and surrounding T2 hyperintensity extending to the ependymal margin of the left lateral ventricle (*B*). The patient had a pathologically proven oligodendroglioma and had undergone proton beam radiation therapy, completed 5 months prior, and several cycles of procarbazine/lomustine. On subsequent imaging, the enhancing nodule had grown (*C*) and there was increased surrounding T2 hyperintensity (*D*). DCE-MR perfusion was performed to help differentiate between tumor progression and radiation necrosis. Region-of-interest interrogation of the enhancing nodule on the Vp map, superimposed on the postcontrast T1 (*E*), demonstrated an elevated plasma volume, approximately double that of normal-appearing white matter. There was also associated elevated permeability (*F, H*). An image from the integrated PET-MR study (*G*) demonstrated that the enhancing nodule had FDG uptake that was greater than adjacent white matter, but less than normal cortex. Subsequent surgical biopsy confirmed radiation-related changes.

of pseudoprogression compared with photon therapy among patients with oligodendroglioma, but not astrocytoma, and pseudoprogression is associated with better progression-free survival.[22] Therefore, these factors have important implications for the interpretation of posttreatment imaging,[33,34] and the diagnostic accuracy of advanced imaging.[35] Interestingly, age and size of the treated lesion were shown to be unrelated to likelihood of pseudoprogresssion.[36] Prospective identification of pseudoprogression is a challenging exercise, and even use of both conventional and advanced imaging techniques may not consistently result in success.[37]

DIFFERENTIATING PSEUDOPROGRESSION FROM TRUE PROGRESSION

Immediate postsurgical imaging should take place within 48 hours postoperatively, in order to avoid postprocedural confounders such as enhancement associated with subacute ischemia.[38] Subsequent follow-up imaging typically takes place after completion of chemoradiation, usually over the course of 6 weeks.

On conventional imaging, enhancement pattern and signal intensity on T2-weighted images are important factors in diagnosing tumor recurrence. Several studies have identified specific enhancement patterns that can aid in elaborating degree of suspicion of true tumor progression. Mullins and colleagues[39] found that involvement of the corpus callosum was most predictive of progression, and that likelihood of tumor progression increased when callosal involvement was seen in combination with multiple enhancing lesions, crossing of the midline, and subependymal spread. Similarly, subependymal enhancement was shown to be predictive of true progression with 93.3% specificity in a retrospective study of 93 patients with GBM undergoing chemoradiation who developed new or increased enhancing mass lesions. However, no features on conventional imaging were found to have high negative predictive value for pseudoprogression.[40] Subependymal enhancement, specifically at a distance from the primary enhancing lesion (>1 cm), was shown to be more common in true progression than pseudoprogression.[41] Focal solid nodular enhancement and solid uniform enhancement with distinct margins was seen in 85% of patients with histopathologically proven tumor recurrence in a group of 51 patients who underwent reoperation after completing chemoradiation.[42]

Increased T2/FLAIR signal is another important qualitative criterion for tumor progression, but can also be seen in the setting of pseudoprogression, secondary to tissue injury or laminar necrosis. However, enhancement in the absence of edema on T2-weighted images is suggestive of pseudoprogression.[43] Signal change extending to cortex and mass effect are more suggestive of tumor progression than pseudoprogression.[44] Increased FLAIR volume and extension beyond the radiation field are also clues to true progression as compared with pseudoprogression.[45] In fact, a postmortem analysis demonstrated that T2-weighted images were most representative of tumor extent compared with postcontrast T1-weighted images when correlated with histopathologic specimens.[46]

Despite heavy reliance on conventional imaging for progression guidelines and attention to subtleties in postcontrast T1 and FLAIR appearance, the sensitivity and specificity of anatomic MR imaging for detection of progression is low. In a recent meta-analysis of 5 studies, including 166 patients, the pooled sensitivity and specificity for anatomic MR imaging was 68% (95% confidence interval [CI] 51–81) and 77% (45–93), respectively, with better performance calculated for advanced imaging techniques (diffusion-weighted imaging [DWI], perfusion-weighted imaging [PWI], and magnetic resonance spectroscopy [MRS]).[37] Ultimately, multimodal assessment might be most productive in differentiating progression from pseudoprogression.[47–51]

MAGNETIC RESONANCE PERFUSION
Perfusion-Weighted Imaging

Three methods are used for PWI, 2 of which rely on the injection of an extrinsic contrast medium (dynamic susceptibility contrast [DSC] and dynamic contrast enhancement [DCE]), and 1 that uses blood as an intrinsic contrast medium (arterial spin labeling [ASL]). In a recent survey conducted by the American Society of Neuroradiology, 151 of 195 institutions endorsed offering perfusion MR imaging and 87% included perfusion as part of the standard brain tumor protocol, with percentage increase to 96% in the evaluation of pseudoprogression[52]; this compared with 48% of a total of 220 health centers across 31 European countries according to a European Society of Neuroradiology survey.[53] DSC was more commonly used than DCE and ASL; and only half of the institutions endorsed quantitative analysis. DSC perfusion, evaluated in 18 studies including 708 patients, had a sensitivity of 87% (82–91) with a specificity of 86% (77–91). DCE-perfusion evaluated in 5 studies including 207 patients had a sensitivity of 92% (73–98) and specificity of 85% (76–92).[52]

Dynamic Susceptibility Contrast

DSC is the most widely used technique for PWI[37]; in a study comparing all 3 perfusion methods, DSC was found to have the best diagnostic performance.[54] DSC relies on T2 and T2* signal changes related to the passage of a paramagnetic contrast agent, and aims at characterizing the hemodynamic properties of the central nervous system microvasculature. A loss of signal versus time curve for every voxel is generated, from which several functional maps are derived. Cerebral blood volume (CBV) is the most commonly used parameter, defined as milliliters of blood per 100 g of brain tissue, and is usually discussed relative to the contralesional brain tissue; this parameter is a surrogate marker for capillary density/neoangiogenesis. Cerebral blood flow (CBF) is the amount of blood in a given volume of tissue per time (mL of blood/100 g brain tissue/min), and is interpreted as the microvascular blood flow in a given region of interest. Mean transit time (MTT) is calculated by dividing CBV by CBF (MTT = CBV/CBF), and is defined as the amount of time it takes for the injected contrast to travel through a defined region or volume of interest. Finally, time to peak is defined as the amount of time it takes for contrast to achieve peak concentration.[55]

Advantages of DSC include its relatively quick and facile execution; limitations include user-dependent calculation of absolute parameter measures and sensitivity to susceptibility-related artifact, particularly at the skull base or in the presence of postoperative hemosiderin deposition. Regional CBV (rCBV) measurements may differ in diagnostic accuracy based on the use of contrast preloading and baseline subtraction techniques.[56] Choice of software package has been shown to bear clinically significant differences in CBV.[57]

In high-grade gliomas, tumor growth leads to neovascularity, increased microvascular density, and slower flow in collateral vasculature, which translates into elevated CBV.[58,59] Multiple studies examining DSC-MR in the setting of posttreatment glioma demonstrate elevated rCBV in the setting of tumor progression.[33,50,54,60–66] Although a recent survey indicated that approximately 50% of surveyed institutions do not process quantitative parameter maps, published studies show that inspection of color maps in the absence of parameter computation does not reliably differentiate progression from psuedoprogression.[67] The challenge in a quantitative approach to DSC-MR is the lack of universal threshold, limiting reproducibility. This is underscored by the wide range of thresholds values for rCBV reported in the literature. For instance, Hu and colleagues[63] demonstrated that an rCBV cutoff value of 0.71 predicted true progression from pseudoprogression with 95.9% accuracy; however, the reported range of rCBV thresholds in the literature range from 0.9 to 2.15 for mean rCBV and 1.49 to 3.10 for maximum rCBV.[68,69] Interestingly, in a meta-analysis examining the utility of DSC perfusion in differentiating progression from pseudoprogression, Wang and colleagues[70] found that differences in threshold values had only a mild effect on individual study accuracy. Other approaches to parameter analysis include rCBV histogram skewness and kurtosis, tumor fractional volume,[68,71,72] parametric response mapping,[73,74] and evaluation of trends over time rather than static computations.[71,75]

Dynamic Contrast Enhancement

DCE is a T1-weighted sequence that usually uses spoiled gradient echo technique, requiring longer acquisition time compared with DSC. Longer acquisition times, ranging from 6 to 10 minutes,[76] are required to characterize the permeability of the blood brain barrier and its relationship to the extracellular extravascular space.[55] Concentration time curves are generated, from which several parameters can be calculated, including Ktrans, the rate of transfer between plasma and extravascular tissue; Kep, the rate of transfer between extravascular tissue and plasma; Ve, the extracellular volume; and Vp, the plasma volume.[77,78] Advantages of DCE include the increased information gained regarding microvascular permeability and blood brain barrier, as well as the technique's decreased sensitivity to susceptibility-related artifact. Disadvantages include the longer scan time, decreased temporal resolution, and differences of opinion regarding ideal pharmacokinetic modeling, which limit comparisons across sites. Compared with DSC, DCE has more limited temporal resolution but improved spatial resolution, and is therefore preferable for lesions with mixed pathology.[16]

The diagnostic accuracy for DCE was shown to be similar to DSC[69] in a meta-analysis performed by van Djiken and colleagues.[37] The expectation, confirmed by several retrospective[79] and prospective[80,81] studies, is that Ktrans and Vp are higher in the setting of true progression compared with pseudoprogression[79,81] and radiation necrosis.[68] Semiquantitative methods using area under the curve (AUC) also have been applied successfully in the evaluation of progression versus pseudoprogression.[82,83] In a retrospective study of 37 patients with GBM and

new/increasing enhancement after treatment, Thomas and colleagues[79] determined that Vp (mean) cutoff less than 3.7 yielded 85% sensitivity and 79% specificity for pseudoprogression and Ktrans (mean) of greater than 3.6 had a 69% sensitivity and 79% specificity for disease progression; however, as with DSC, universal thresholds have not been established.[84]

Arterial Spin Labeling

ASL is a technique that uses a series of short radiofrequency pulses to label endogenous protons in arterial blood.[85] CBF is calculated based on the difference in signal between baseline images and the magnetically labeled images, and can be applied using a pseudocontinuous or pulsed technique.[86] Labeling time is approximately 2 to 4 seconds, followed by a 1.5-second to 2.0-second delay, after which signal is acquired by using fast spin echo or gradient echo technique.[77,78] The calculated parameter of interest is CBF, which has been shown to correlate well with rCBV generated using DCE technique, but, unlike DCE, leakage correction is not required.[86] Because of the intrinsically low signal to noise, ASL scan times are longer and therefore prone to motion artifact.[85,87] Moreover, complexity of ASL flow calculations make ASL a less popular perfusion technique.[87] Studies have demonstrated the utility of ASL as both an independent perfusion method[55] and as an adjunct to other perfusion methods such as DSC[88] in differentiating between progression and pseudoprogression; however, this method is less frequently used for reasons discussed previously.

DIFFUSION
Diffusion-Weighted Imaging

DWI is an MR imaging technique sensitive to the molecular motion of water through the addition of 2 identical diffusion gradients, one on each side of a 180° refocusing pulse[89]; increased cellularity in the setting of high-grade glioma confers high microscopic tissue organization, and is detected as reduced diffusion.[77] Apparent diffusion coefficient (ADC), a measure of water diffusivity, has therefore been used in the differentiation of tumor progression from pseudoprogression.[66,89–93]

DWI can be used as both a qualitative[90,93] and quantitative[91,94,95] imaging tool in differentiating progression from pseudoprogression. For instance, on the basis of visual inspection alone, Lee and colleagues[90] found that in a group of 22 patients with GBM treated with chemoradiation, the progression group showed a higher incidence of homogeneous or multifocal high signal intensity on diffusion-weighted images, whereas only peripheral hyperintensity or no high signal intensity was more frequently observed in the pseudoprogression group. Using a quantitative approach, multiple studies have shown that mean ADC values are lower in patients with true progression as compared with pseudoprogression[41,90,92,94]; relative similarity in thresholds has been demonstrated between studies.[91,92] ADC values are particularly useful in the setting of nonenhancing T2/FLAIR hyperintensity, as low ADC values have been shown to precede the appearance of enhancing, viable tumor by a median of 3 months in patients undergoing treatment for GBM.[96] In addition to qualitative diffusion features and mean ADC values, cumulative ADC histogram analysis has been shown to aid in the differentiation of true progression from pseudoprogression,[97–99] as have voxel-wise approaches using parametric response maps[95] and functional diffusion maps.[100]

Diffusion Tensor Imaging

Diffusion tensor imaging (DTI) is an MR imaging technique that is sensitive to not only the degree but the direction of water diffusion. The technique applies at least 6 noncollinear directions of diffusion sensitization; the number of diffusion sensitizing directions can vary from 6 to 256.[101] Multiple quantitative parameters can be calculated, including fractional anisotropy (FA), which is a summary measure reflecting the overall directional coherence of water.

Studies using DTI in posttreatment monitoring show mixed interpretation of diffusion parameters. Although one might expect higher FA in areas of true tumor progression compared with pseudoprogression, ostensibly due to increased cellularity and therefore tissue organization expected in high-grade glioma, the limited number of studies applying DTI in the setting of treatment response have shown inconsistent results, with studies showing no difference in FA,[102,103] higher FA,[70] and lower FA[104] values in true progression compared with pseudoprogression.

Magnetic Resonance Spectroscopy

MRS is a technique that identifies and quantifies particular metabolites in a lesion of interest. MRS can be performed using multi-voxel or single-voxel techniques, to generate a plot of signal to frequency, expressed in parts per million.[77,105,106] Clinically relevant metabolites include N-acetylaspartate (NAA), a marker of neuronal viability; total choline (tCho), a marker of cell membrane turnover/cellular proliferation; total creatine (tCr), an

energy metabolite; lactate, a product of anaerobic glycolytic metabolism; and lipid (triglycerides), a marker of necrosis.[77,106] Given its stable concentration, creatine is used as the reference for report of the metabolites of interest,[107] and typically high-grade gliomas are characterized by elevation of tCho and decrease in NAA.[108–111]

Limitations of MRS are multiple. Single-voxel approaches are prone to partial volume effects,[112] and there is limited ability to detect smaller lesions. Because of low metabolite concentrations, multiple acquisitions are required necessitating long scan times and, finally, there is the technical onus of eliminating contamination from adjacent tissues, such as scalp and ventricle.[37] Nevertheless, in a pooled meta-analysis of 9 studies including 203 patients, van Dijken and colleagues[37] found that MRS had the highest accuracy in response evaluation compared with conventional MR imaging, DWI, and perfusion MR imaging, with sensitivity of spectroscopy reported at 91% (79–97) and specificity reported at 95% (65–99).

MRS is a useful tool in determining progression from pseudoprogression. In a longitudinal study, Sawlani and colleagues[113] used single-voxel MRS to show elevation of lipid peaks and decrease in tCho/NAA ratios in patients with pseudoprogression, whereas elevated Cho and elevated tCho/NAA ratio were seen in patients with true progression. In a prospective study of 24 patients with GBM, significant differences in MRS data were recorded for patients with progression and pseudoprogression, with ideal institutional recurrence thresholds established as tNAA $\leq$1.5 mM, tCho/tNAA $\geq$1.4 (sensitivity 100%, specificity 91.7%), tNAA/Cr $\leq$0.7[91]; the investigators subsequently validated these thresholds, and concluded that GBM relapse was characterized by the tCho/tNAA ratio $\geq$1.3 with sensitivity of 100% and specificity of 94.7% (P<.001).[92] However, some studies have shown that Cho and NAA are increased in both progression and pseudoprogression, particularly in the early post-radiation time point.[114] Recently, 2-hydroxyglutarate was noted to accumulate in tumors with the IDH mutation,[115] and this metabolite can be used to monitor response to treatment in IDH-mutated gliomas.[116]

PET with Fludeoxyglucose

The most widely used PET tracer is, 2-(18F) fluoro-2-deoxy-D-glucose (FDG), a glucose analog incorporated into glycolytic metabolism; FDG-PET is used to monitor treatment response in glioblastoma.[117–120] Standardized uptake values represent the ratio of radiotracer activity in tissue relative to the injected dose per kilogram of body weight. Limitations to FDG-PET include physiologic uptake in normal brain parenchyma, constraining evaluation of small lesions, in addition to the observation that some high-grade gliomas may have decreased FDG uptake, creating a confusing clinical picture.[121]

A meta-analysis of 18F-FDG-PET utility in detecting recurrence in glioma revealed pooled sensitivity of 0.77 (95% CI, 0.66–0.85) and specificity of 0.78 (95% CI, 0.54–0.91).[122] A wide range of standardized uptake value (SUV) cutoff values for detection of glioma recurrence are reported in the literature, ranging from 1.3 to 1.5 relative to normal white matter, 0.5 to 1.05 relative to normal gray matter, and 1.3 to 1.35 for a mirror-image location as a reference,[106] with equally varying degrees of sensitivity and specificity.[123]

The utility of radiolabeled amino acid PET tracers in the posttreatment setting has also been explored. 11C–MET PET/MR imaging has been shown to have greater sensitivity, specificity and AUC compared with FDG-PET[124] and compared with MR imaging alone.[122,125] However, 11C-MET has a short half-life and therefore requires an on-site cyclotron, limiting its practical use. O-(2–18FFluoroethyl)- L-tyrosine (18F-FET) has a longer half-life than 11C-MET, and has been similarly applied in treatment monitoring.[126–130] Disadvantages of 18F-FET include slower renal elimination, resulting in increased residual tracer in the blood pool and, therefore, nonspecific tracer uptake.[131]

PSEUDOPROGRESSION IN IMMUNOTHERAPY

In the setting of immunotherapy, increase in size of a treated lesion may reflect a localized inflammatory response induced by immunotherapy and apparent new, enhancing lesions may represent immune response in previously infiltrative, nonenhancing disease. Delayed response and/or a "flare phenomenon" may occur,[132,133] and a number of studies have been performed to explore the associated perfusion[134,135] and diffusion[135,136] changes. Application of MRS to treatment response in immunotherapy also has been explored,[137] and has been shown to aid in identification of pseudoprogression in the setting of new lesion enhancement. Because lipid is a substrate of natural killer T cells, a lipid peak on MRS may be seen in the setting of immunotherapy response.[77,138] The application of FDG-PET and ASL have been less well-explored, and remain important potential avenues for future research efforts.

PSEUDORESPONSE

Whereas pseudoprogression typically occurs in the setting of administration of radiation and an alkylating agent, pseudoresponse occurs in the setting of antiangiogenic therapy. Glioblastoma is a highly vascular tumor that depends on angiogenesis for growth, with upregulation of several proangiogenic factors, including VEGF, hepatocyte growth factor, fibroblast growth factor, platelet-derived growth factor, angiopoietins, and IL-8,[139] resulting in disorganized vasculature with abnormalities in endothelial wall, pericyte coverage, and basement membrane.[140] Bevacizumab is a humanized monoclonal antibody that targets and binds VEGF-A, a highly expressed proangiogenic factor in brain tumors.[139] By targeting VEGF, normalization of tumor vasculature occurs with decrease in vessel size and permeability. This alteration in vasculature is believed to improve delivery of chemotherapy and/or radiation therapy.[141]

Imaging findings after anti-VEGF therapy include decreased contrast enhancement, edema, and permeability as early as 1 day after initiation of therapy.[141] Radiologic response rates are high, ranging from 25% to 60%.[1,2] Despite remarkable imaging response following bevacizumab administration, there has been no proven substantial benefit in overall survival. Bevacizumab, however, has been shown to improve progression-free survival with decreased patient dependence on steroid treatment.[142] A large fraction of patients who initially demonstrate radiographic response eventually develop progressive disease in the form of worsening, nonenhancing T2 signal hyperintensity on T2 FLAIR sequences.[143] Although presence of increased T2 FLAIR signal in nonenhancing tumor during antiangiogenic therapy has been shown to be associated with a higher risk of death, the usage of T2 FLAIR monitoring has been controversial given variability in interpretation.[144]

Several imaging methods have been investigated to distinguish true response from pseudoresponse in the setting of antiangiogenic therapy. The utility of perfusion imaging has been explored with equivocal results. Stadlbauer and colleagues[145] pointed out the limitation of DSC perfusion, because both normal brain parenchyma and tumor exhibit decreased perfusion following bevacizumab administration. Other studies have demonstrated the utility of DSC perfusion in detecting decrease in permeability following antiangiogenic therapy, which correlated with overall survival or progression-free survival.[146,147]

Although ADC value is helpful in differentiating true progression from pseudoprogression, ADC values may be of limited usefulness in evaluating pseudoresponse. A recent study of ADC values in patients on bevacizumab demonstrated normalization of ADC values following initiation of treatment that persisted even when progressive disease was reported.[148] However, preantiangiogenic treatment ADC values at a threshold of greater than 1.24 μm^2/ms have been shown to predict improved overall survival in patients with recurrent glioblastoma.[149]

More recently, amino acid PET has shown promising ability to improve identification of viable tumor by detecting the tumor's demand for carbon. A case report cited the ability of radiolabeled amino acid 18F-FET PET to detect progressive tumors earlier in patients treated with bevacizumab.[150] Another study, investigating the use of radiolabeled 3,4-dihydroxy-6-[18F]-fluoro-L-phenylalanine (18F-FDOPA) PET found that

metabolic tumor volumes were predictive of treatment response and overall survival as early as 2 weeks following the initiation of bevacizumab.[151] Fig. 3 illustrates the temporal progression of imaging findings of a glioblastoma treated with bevacizumab after tumor progression.

RADIATION NECROSIS

Radiation necrosis and pseudoprogression are often thought of as 2 opposite extremes along the spectrum of radiation-induced injury. The terms are often interchanged, and several studies examining progression versus "treatment-related change" refer to pseudoprogression and radiation necrosis as a single collective entity.[49,54,152–154] However, pseudoprogression and radiation necrosis are, in fact, distinct in timing, pathomechanism, histopathology, and prognosis.

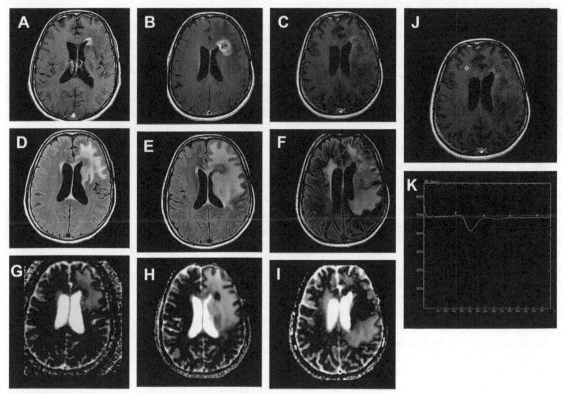

Fig. 3. Pseudoresponse. Axial postcontrast T1 (*A–C*), T2 FLAIR (*D–F*), and corresponding ADC maps showing the temporal progression of imaging findings of a glioblastoma that progressed and was subsequently treated with bevacizumab. The initial imaging demonstrated an area of enhancement along the left frontal horn (*A*), with surrounding T2 hyperintensity (*D*) likely representing a combination of infiltrative tumor, vasogenic edema, and/or treatment-related gliosis. A small focus of ADC hypointensity was also noted (*G*). A month later, both the enhancement (*B*) and T2 hyperintensity (*E*) progressed, with associated expansion of the area of ADC hypointensity (*H*), possibly reflecting hypercellular tumor. Bevacizumab therapy was started immediately after this scan. Two months later, the enhancement had decreased significantly (*C*), giving the appearance of a response to therapy. However, the area of heterogeneous T2 hyperintensity (*F*) and ADC hypointensity (*I*) further expanded. This was biopsy-proven to be viable tumor. Of note, DSC-MR perfusion was misleading by demonstrating no elevated CBV in the area of enhancement (*J*, *K*), likely given the antiangiogenic effect of the bevacizumab.

Pseudoprogression typically occurs within weeks to months after treatment, whereas radiation necrosis typically occurs 9 to 12 months after treatment and can occur up to several years later; new areas of contrast enhancement are typically bounded by the initial radiation field.[44] In pseudoprogression, vasodilation, perturbations in the blood brain barrier, and vasogenic edema lead to transient effects, whereas more severe injury in radiation necrosis related to oligodendrocyte injury, autoimmune mechanisms, and endothelial cell death leads to more irreversible fibrinoid necrosis, fibrosis, reactive gliosis, demyelination, and vascular hyalinization.[10,26,37] Perhaps the most important distinction between the two is that patients with pseudoprogression have a more favorable prognosis, whereas patients with radiation necrosis experience more profound neurologic decline and ultimately have a worse prognosis.[16] The frequency of radiation necrosis is reported anywhere from 5% to 25%, with risk proportionate to radiation dose,[16,155,156] with the 1p/19q codeletion shown to be a significant risk factor.[157] Treatment options for radiation necrosis include bevacizumab, anticoagulation, hyperbaric oxygen therapy, vitamin E, and laser interstitial thermal therapy.[10]

On conventional imaging, several imaging features are suggestive of radiation necrosis compared with progression. Radiation necrosis typically involves the periventricular white matter within or adjacent to the radiation field, due to its tenuous blood supply,[16] but can occur in a contralesional and multifocal distribution as well.[158] Internal enhancement patterns, described as "Swiss-cheese" or "soap-bubble," have been shown to be more typical of radiation necrosis,[158] as has the presence of diffuse, "meshlike enhancement" or peripheral enhancement with "feathery" margins.[42,159] On T2-weighted imaging, the central necrotic component will have high signal, whereas the solid component will have relatively lower signal.

Advanced imaging techniques available for differentiation between radiation necrosis and progression are similar to those applied in the early posttreatment period in evaluating for pseudoprogression[48,160] and include DWI,[161,162] PWI,[163] including DSC,[152,164] DCE,[154,165] and ASL,[166] MRS,[167–170] and PET.[171] In general, true progression will exhibit increased perfusion,[152,164,172] elevated rCBV,[173] lower ADC values on DWI,[41,104,161,172] higher Cho/Cr (choline/creatine) and Cho/NAA (choline/N-acetyl aspartate) ratios and lower NAA/Cr ratios,[77,160] and increased SUV uptake in true progression compared with radiation necrosis. The presence of a lipid peak is suggestive of radiation necrosis[77]; multivoxel MRS has been shown to be superior in diagnostic accuracy to single-voxel MRS, particularly in the setting of mixed pathology lesions.[174] There have been mixed results in terms of MRS and PET accuracy, and meta-analyses have shown moderate sensitivity and specificity for MRS,[175] 18F-FDG, and 11C-MET PET[122] in differentiating between progression and radiation necrosis. Kim and colleagues found no difference between recurrence and necrosis groups using 18F-FDG and 11C-MET PET.[173] FDG-PET may have more limited utility than perfusion and DWI in differentiation of tumor progression from radiation necrosis,[176] and although MRS is highly accurate in differentiating between high-grade and low-grade gliomas, it may be less useful in differentiating between true progression and radiation necrosis.[177]

SUMMARY

Treatment response assessment in glioblastoma is important to management decisions and legitimacy of clinical trials. The RANO criteria are the most widely used guidelines in glioma response, but new enhancement seen within the radiation field during the first 12 weeks after treatment is difficult to definitively classify as true progression. Several patterns of enhancement and T2 signal are suggestive of pseudoprogression and radiation necrosis; ultimately, a multimodality approach including advanced imaging has been shown to result in greatest diagnostic accuracy. Pseudoresponse is difficult to discriminate from true response, given that the antiangiogenic effect has been shown to suppress imaging features suggestive of disease progression, even in the absence of increased overall survival. Knowledge of the strengths and limitations of various imaging techniques described previously can help the radiologist to synthesize and integrate provided imaging and clinical data to develop a more evidence-based assessment of true disease progression.

REFERENCES

1. Ostrom QT, Gittleman H, Truitt G, et al. CBTRUS statistical report: primary brain and other central nervous system tumors diagnosed in the United States in 2011–2015. Neuro Oncol 2018; 20(suppl_4):iv1–86.
2. Stupp R, Mason WP, Van Den Bent MJ, et al. Radiotherapy plus concomitant and adjuvant temozolomide for glioblastoma. N Engl J Med 2005; 352(10):987–96.

3. Khasraw M, Ameratunga MS, Grant R, et al. Antiangiogenic therapy for high-grade glioma. Cochrane Database Syst Rev 2014;(9):CD008218.

4. Domingo-Musibay E, Galanis E. What next for newly diagnosed glioblastoma? Future Oncol 2015;11(24):3273–83.

5. Dusek L, Muzik J, Maluskova D, et al. Cancer incidence and mortality in the Czech Republic. Klin Onkol 2014;27(6):406–23.

6. Weathers S-P, Gilbert MR. Current challenges in designing GBM trials for immunotherapy. J Neurooncol 2015;123(3):331–7.

7. Weinberg BD, Gore A, Shu H-KG, et al. Management-based structured reporting of posttreatment glioma response with the brain tumor reporting and data system. J Am Coll Radiol 2018;15(5):767–71.

8. Levin VA, Crafts DC, Norman DM, et al. Criteria for evaluating patients undergoing chemotherapy for malignant brain tumors. J Neurosurg 1977;47(3):329–35.

9. Macdonald DR, Cascino TL, Schold SC Jr, et al. Response criteria for phase II studies of supratentorial malignant glioma. J Clin Oncol 1990;8(7):1277–80.

10. Delgado-Lopez P, Corrales-Garcia E. Survival in glioblastoma: a review on the impact of treatment modalities. Clin Transl Oncol 2016;18(11):1062–71.

11. Eisenhauer EA, Therasse P, Bogaerts J, et al. New response evaluation criteria in solid tumours: revised RECIST guideline (version 1.1). Eur J Cancer 2009;45(2):228–47.

12. Wen PY, Macdonald DR, Reardon DA, et al. Updated response assessment criteria for high-grade gliomas: response assessment in neuro-oncology working group. J Clin Oncol 2010;28(11):1963–72.

13. Okada H, Weller M, Huang R, et al. Immunotherapy response assessment in neuro-oncology: a report of the RANO working group. Lancet Oncol 2015;16(15):e534–42.

14. Okada H, Kohanbash G, Zhu X, et al. Immunotherapeutic approaches for glioma. Crit Rev Immunol 2009;29(1):1–42.

15. Ellingson BM, Wen PY, Cloughesy TF. Modified criteria for radiographic response assessment in glioblastoma clinical trials. Neurotherapeutics 2017;14(2):307–20.

16. Brandsma D, Stalpers L, Taal W, et al. Clinical features, mechanisms, and management of pseudoprogression in malignant gliomas. Lancet Oncol 2008;9(5):453–61.

17. Chaskis C, Neyns B, Michotte A, et al. Pseudoprogression after radiotherapy with concurrent temozolomide for high-grade glioma: clinical observations and working recommendations. Surg Neurol 2009;72(4):423–8.

18. Carceller F, Mandeville H, Mackinnon AD, et al. Facing pseudoprogression after radiotherapy in low grade gliomas. Transl Cancer Res 2017;6(Suppl 2):S254–8.

19. van West SE, de Bruin HG, van de Langerijt B, et al. Incidence of pseudoprogression in low-grade gliomas treated with radiotherapy. Neuro Oncol 2017;19(5):719–25.

20. Clarke JL, Chang S. Pseudoprogression and pseudoresponse: challenges in brain tumor imaging. Curr Neurol Neurosci Rep 2009;9(3):241–6.

21. Dworkin M, Mehan W, Niemierko A, et al. Increase of pseudoprogression and other treatment related effects in low-grade glioma patients treated with proton radiation and temozolomide. J Neurooncol 2019;142(1):69–77.

22. Bronk JK, Guha-Thakurta N, Allen PK, et al. Analysis of pseudoprogression after proton or photon therapy of 99 patients with low grade and anaplastic glioma. Clin Transl Radiat Oncol 2018;9:30–4.

23. De Wit M, De Bruin H, Eijkenboom W, et al. Immediate post-radiotherapy changes in malignant glioma can mimic tumor progression. Neurology 2004;63(3):535–7.

24. Chamberlain MC, Glantz MJ, Chalmers L, et al. Early necrosis following concurrent Temodar and radiotherapy in patients with glioblastoma. J Neurooncol 2007;82(1):81–3.

25. Fatterpekar GM, Galheigo D, Narayana A, et al. Treatment-related change versus tumor recurrence in high-grade gliomas: a diagnostic conundrum—use of dynamic susceptibility contrast-enhanced (DSC) perfusion MRI. AJR Am J Roentgenol 2012;198(1):19–26.

26. Melguizo-Gavilanes I, Bruner JM, Guha-Thakurta N, et al. Characterization of pseudoprogression in patients with glioblastoma: is histology the gold standard? J Neurooncol 2015;123(1):141–50.

27. Weller M, Tabatabai G, Kästner B, et al. MGMT promoter methylation is a strong prognostic biomarker for benefit from dose-intensified temozolomide re-challenge in progressive glioblastoma: the DIRECTOR trial. Clin Cancer Res 2015;21(9):2057–64.

28. Brandes AA, Tosoni A, Franceschi E, et al. Recurrence pattern after temozolomide concomitant with and adjuvant to radiotherapy in newly diagnosed patients with glioblastoma: correlation with MGMT promoter methylation status. J Clin Oncol 2009;27(8):1275–9.

29. Hegi ME, Diserens A-C, Gorlia T, et al. MGMT gene silencing and benefit from temozolomide in glioblastoma. N Engl J Med 2005;352(10):997–1003.

30. Li H, Li J, Cheng G, et al. IDH mutation and MGMT promoter methylation are associated with the pseudoprogression and improved prognosis of

glioblastoma multiforme patients who have undergone concurrent and adjuvant temozolomide-based chemoradiotherapy. Clin Neurol Neurosurg 2016;151:31–6.

31. Brandes AA, Franceschi E, Tosoni A, et al. MGMT promoter methylation status can predict the incidence and outcome of pseudoprogression after concomitant radiochemotherapy in newly diagnosed glioblastoma patients. J Clin Oncol 2008; 26(13):2192–7.

32. Motegi H, Kamoshima Y, Terasaka S, et al. IDH1 mutation as a potential novel biomarker for distinguishing pseudoprogression from true progression in patients with glioblastoma treated with temozolomide and radiotherapy. Brain Tumor Pathol 2013; 30(2):67–72.

33. Kong D-S, Kim S, Kim E-H, et al. Diagnostic dilemma of pseudoprogression in the treatment of newly diagnosed glioblastomas: the role of assessing relative cerebral blood flow volume and oxygen-6-methylguanine-DNA methyltransferase promoter methylation status. AJNR Am J Neuroradiol 2011;32(2):382–7.

34. Drabycz S, Roldán G, De Robles P, et al. An analysis of image texture, tumor location, and MGMT promoter methylation in glioblastoma using magnetic resonance imaging. Neuroimage 2010;49(2): 1398–405.

35. Yoon RG, Kim HS, Paik W, et al. Different diagnostic values of imaging parameters to predict pseudoprogression in glioblastoma subgroups stratified by MGMT promoter methylation. Eur Radiol 2017; 27(1):255–66.

36. Taal W, Brandsma D, De Bruin H, et al. The incidence of pseudo-progression in a cohort of malignant glioma patients treated with chemo-radiation with temozolomide. J Clin Oncol 2007;25(18_suppl):2009.

37. van Dijken BR, van Laar PJ, Holtman GA, et al. Diagnostic accuracy of magnetic resonance imaging techniques for treatment response evaluation in patients with high-grade glioma, a systematic review and meta-analysis. Eur Radiol 2017;27(10): 4129–44.

38. Henegar MM, Moran CJ, Silbergeld DL. Early postoperative magnetic resonance imaging following nonneoplastic cortical resection. J Neurosurg 1996;84(2):174–9.

39. Mullins ME, Barest GD, Schaefer PW, et al. Radiation necrosis versus glioma recurrence: conventional MR imaging clues to diagnosis. AJNR Am J Neuroradiol 2005;26(8):1967–72.

40. Young R, Gupta A, Shah A, et al. Potential utility of conventional MRI signs in diagnosing pseudoprogression in glioblastoma. Neurology 2011;76(22): 1918–24.

41. Yoo R-E, Choi S, Kim T, et al. Independent poor prognostic factors for true progression after radiation therapy and concomitant temozolomide in patients with glioblastoma: subependymal enhancement and low ADC value. AJNR Am J Neuroradiol 2015;36(10):1846–52.

42. Reddy K, Westerly D, Chen C. MRI patterns of T 1 enhancing radiation necrosis versus tumour recurrence in high-grade gliomas. J Med Imaging Radiat Oncol 2013;57(3):349–55.

43. Kleinberg L, Yoon G, Weingart JD, et al. Imaging after GliaSite brachytherapy: prognostic MRI indicators of disease control and recurrence. Int J Radiat Oncol Biol Phys 2009;75(5): 1385–91.

44. Dalesandro MF, Andre JB. Posttreatment evaluation of brain gliomas. Neuroimage Clin 2016; 26(4):581–99.

45. Abel R, Jones J, Mandelin P, et al. Distinguishing pseudoprogression from true progression by FLAIR volumetric characteristics compared to 45 Gy isodose volumes in treated glioblastoma patients. Int J Radiat Oncol Biol Phys 2012;84(3): S275.

46. Johnson PC, Hunt SJ, Drayer BP. Human cerebral gliomas: correlation of postmortem MR imaging and neuropathologic findings. Radiology 1989; 170(1):211–7.

47. Liu Z-C, Yan L-F, Hu Y-C, et al. Combination of IVIM-DWI and 3D-ASL for differentiating true progression from pseudoprogression of Glioblastoma multiforme after concurrent chemoradiotherapy: study protocol of a prospective diagnostic trial. BMC Med Imaging 2017;17(1):10.

48. Matsusue E, Fink JR, Rockhill JK, et al. Distinction between glioma progression and post-radiation change by combined physiologic MR imaging. Neuroradiology 2010;52(4):297–306.

49. Kim HS, Goh MJ, Kim N, et al. Which combination of MR imaging modalities is best for predicting recurrent glioblastoma? Study of diagnostic accuracy and reproducibility. Radiology 2014;273(3): 831–43.

50. Cha J, Kim ST, Kim H-J, et al. Differentiation of tumor progression from pseudoprogression in patients with posttreatment glioblastoma using multiparametric histogram analysis. AJNR Am J Neuroradiol 2014;35(7):1309–17.

51. Suh CH, Kim HS, Jung SC, et al. Multiparametric MRI as a potential surrogate endpoint for decision-making in early treatment response following concurrent chemoradiotherapy in patients with newly diagnosed glioblastoma: a systematic review and meta-analysis. Eur Radiol 2018;28(6):2628–38.

52. Dickerson E, Srinivasan A. Multicenter survey of current practice patterns in perfusion MRI in neuroradiology: why, when, and how is it performed? AJR Am J Roentgenol 2016;207(2):406–10.

53. Thust S, Heiland S, Falini A, et al. Glioma imaging in Europe: a survey of 220 centres and recommendations for best clinical practice. Eur Radiol 2018; 28(8):3306–17.

54. Seeger A, Braun C, Skardelly M, et al. Comparison of three different MR perfusion techniques and MR spectroscopy for multiparametric assessment in distinguishing recurrent high-grade gliomas from stable disease. Acad Radiol 2013;20(12):1557–65.

55. McGehee BE, Pollock JM, Maldjian JA. Brain perfusion imaging: how does it work and what should I use? J Magn Reson Imaging 2012;36(6):1257–72.

56. Hu LS, Baxter L, Pinnaduwage D, et al. Optimized preload leakage-correction methods to improve the diagnostic accuracy of dynamic susceptibility-weighted contrast-enhanced perfusion MR imaging in posttreatment gliomas. AJNR Am J Neuroradiol 2010;31(1):40–8.

57. Kelm ZS, Korfiatis PD, Lingineni RK, et al. Variability and accuracy of different software packages for dynamic susceptibility contrast magnetic resonance imaging for distinguishing glioblastoma progression from pseudoprogression. J Med Imaging 2015;2(2):026001.

58. Aronen HJ, Gazit IE, Louis DN, et al. Cerebral blood volume maps of gliomas: comparison with tumor grade and histologic findings. Radiology 1994;191(1):41–51.

59. Sood S, Gupta A, Tsiouris AJ. Advanced magnetic resonance techniques in neuroimaging: diffusion, spectroscopy, and perfusion. Semin Roentgenol 2010;45(2):137–46.

60. Dandois V, Rommel D, Renard L, et al. Substitution of 11C-methionine PET by perfusion MRI during the follow-up of treated high-grade gliomas: preliminary results in clinical practice. J Neuroradiol 2010;37(2):89–97.

61. Di Costanzo A, Scarabino T, Trojsi F, et al. Recurrent glioblastoma multiforme versus radiation injury: a multiparametric 3-T MR approach. Radiol Med 2014;119(8):616–24.

62. Heidemans-Hazelaar C, Van der Kallen B, de Kanter AV, et al. perfusion MR in differentiating between tumor-progression and pseudo-progression in recurrent glioblastoma multiforme: O. 02. Neuro Oncol 2010;12(3):1.

63. Hu LS, Baxter L, Smith K, et al. Relative cerebral blood volume values to differentiate high-grade glioma recurrence from posttreatment radiation effect: direct correlation between image-guided tissue histopathology and localized dynamic susceptibility-weighted contrast-enhanced perfusion MR imaging measurements. AJNR Am J Neuroradiol 2009;30(3):552–8.

64. Mangla R, Singh G, Ziegelitz D, et al. Changes in relative cerebral blood volume 1 month after radiation-temozolomide therapy can help predict overall survival in patients with glioblastoma. Radiology 2010;256(2):575–84.

65. Sugahara T, Korogi Y, Tomiguchi S, et al. Posttherapeutic intraaxial brain tumor: the value of perfusion-sensitive contrast-enhanced MR imaging for differentiating tumor recurrence from nonneoplastic contrast-enhancing tissue. AJNR Am J Neuroradiol 2000;21(5):901–9.

66. Prager A, Martinez N, Beal K, et al. Diffusion and perfusion MRI to differentiate treatment-related changes including pseudoprogression from recurrent tumors in high-grade gliomas with histopathologic evidence. AJNR Am J Neuroradiol 2015; 36(5):877–85.

67. Kerkhof M, Tans PL, Hagenbeek RE, et al. Visual inspection of MR relative cerebral blood volume maps has limited value for distinguishing progression from pseudoprogression in glioblastoma multiforme patients. CNS Oncol 2017;6(04): 297–306.

68. Hyare H, Thust S, Rees J. Advanced MRI techniques in the monitoring of treatment of gliomas. Curr Treat Options Neurol 2017;19(3):11.

69. Patel P, Baradaran H, Delgado D, et al. MR perfusion-weighted imaging in the evaluation of high-grade gliomas after treatment: a systematic review and meta-analysis. Neuro Oncol 2016; 19(1):118–27.

70. Wang Q, Zhang H, Zhang J, et al. The diagnostic performance of magnetic resonance spectroscopy in differentiating high-from low-grade gliomas: a systematic review and meta-analysis. Eur Radiol 2016;26(8):2670–84.

71. Baek HJ, Kim HS, Kim N, et al. Percent change of perfusion skewness and kurtosis: a potential imaging biomarker for early treatment response in patients with newly diagnosed glioblastomas. Radiology 2012;264(3):834–43.

72. Hu LS, Eschbacher JM, Heiserman JE, et al. Reevaluating the imaging definition of tumor progression: perfusion MRI quantifies recurrent glioblastoma tumor fraction, pseudoprogression, and radiation necrosis to predict survival. Neuro Oncol 2012;14(7):919–30.

73. Tsien C, Galbán CJ, Chenevert TL, et al. Parametric response map as an imaging biomarker to distinguish progression from pseudoprogression in high-grade glioma. J Clin Oncol 2010;28(13):2293.

74. Galbán CJ, Chenevert TL, Meyer CR, et al. The parametric response map is an imaging biomarker for early cancer treatment outcome. Nat Med 2009; 15(5):572.

75. Boxerman JL, Ellingson BM, Jeyapalan S, et al. Longitudinal DSC-MRI for distinguishing tumor recurrence from pseudoprogression in patients with a high-grade glioma. Am J Clin Oncol 2017; 40(3):228–34.

76. Paldino MJ, Barboriak DP. Fundamentals of quantitative dynamic contrast-enhanced MR imaging. Magn Reson Imaging Clin N Am 2009;17(2): 277–89.

77. Aquino D, Gioppo A, Finocchiaro G, et al. MRI in glioma immunotherapy: evidence, pitfalls, and perspectives. J Immunol Res 2017;2017:5813951.

78. van Dijken BR, van Laar PJ, Smits M, et al. Perfusion MRI in treatment evaluation of glioblastomas: Clinical relevance of current and future techniques. J Magn Reson Imaging 2019;49(1):11–22.

79. Thomas AA, Arevalo-Perez J, Kaley T, et al. Dynamic contrast enhanced T1 MRI perfusion differentiates pseudoprogression from recurrent glioblastoma. J Neurooncol 2015;125(1):183–90.

80. Bisdas S, Naegele T, Ritz R, et al. Distinguishing recurrent high-grade gliomas from radiation injury: a pilot study using dynamic contrast-enhanced MR imaging. Acad Radiol 2011;18(5):575–83.

81. Yun TJ, Park C-K, Kim TM, et al. Glioblastoma treated with concurrent radiation therapy and temozolomide chemotherapy: differentiation of true progression from pseudoprogression with quantitative dynamic contrast-enhanced MR imaging. Radiology 2015;274(3):830–40.

82. Chung WJ, Kim HS, Kim N, et al. Recurrent glioblastoma: optimum area under the curve method derived from dynamic contrast-enhanced T1-weighted perfusion MR imaging. Radiology 2013; 269(2):561–8.

83. Suh C, Kim H, Choi Y, et al. Prediction of pseudoprogression in patients with glioblastomas using the initial and final area under the curves ratio derived from dynamic contrast-enhanced T1-weighted perfusion MR imaging. AJNR Am J Neuroradiol 2013;34(12):2278–86.

84. Heo YJ, Kim HS, Park JE, et al. Uninterpretable dynamic susceptibility contrast-enhanced perfusion MR images in patients with post-treatment glioblastomas: cross-validation of alternative imaging options. PLoS One 2015;10(8):e0136380.

85. Williams DS, Detre JA, Leigh JS, et al. Magnetic resonance imaging of perfusion using spin inversion of arterial water. Proc Natl Acad Sci U S A 1992;89(1):212–6.

86. Telischak NA, Detre JA, Zaharchuk G. Arterial spin labeling MRI: clinical applications in the brain. J Magn Reson Imaging 2015;41(5):1165–80.

87. Petersen E, Zimine I, Ho YL, et al. Non-invasive measurement of perfusion: a critical review of arterial spin labelling techniques. Br J Radiol 2006; 79(944):688–701.

88. Choi YJ, Kim HS, Jahng G-H, et al. Pseudoprogression in patients with glioblastoma: added value of arterial spin labeling to dynamic susceptibility contrast perfusion MR imaging. Acta Radiol 2013; 54(4):448–54.

89. Schmainda KM. Diffusion-weighted MRI as a biomarker for treatment response in glioma. CNS Oncol 2012;1(2):169–80.

90. Lee WJ, Choi SH, Park C-K, et al. Diffusion-weighted MR imaging for the differentiation of true progression from pseudoprogression following concomitant radiotherapy with temozolomide in patients with newly diagnosed high-grade gliomas. Acad Radiol 2012;19(11):1353–61.

91. Bulik M, Kazda T, Slampa P, et al. The diagnostic ability of follow-up imaging biomarkers after treatment of glioblastoma in the temozolomide era: implications from proton MR spectroscopy and apparent diffusion coefficient mapping. Biomed Res Int 2015;2015:641023.

92. Kazda T, Bulik M, Pospisil P, et al. Advanced MRI increases the diagnostic accuracy of recurrent glioblastoma: single institution thresholds and validation of MR spectroscopy and diffusion weighted MR imaging. Neuroimage Clin 2016;11:316–21.

93. Asao C, Korogi Y, Kitajima M, et al. Diffusion-weighted imaging of radiation-induced brain injury for differentiation from tumor recurrence. AJNR Am J Neuroradiol 2005;26(6):1455–60.

94. Hein PA, Eskey CJ, Dunn JF, et al. Diffusion-weighted imaging in the follow-up of treated high-grade gliomas: tumor recurrence versus radiation injury. AJNR Am J Neuroradiol 2004;25(2):201–9.

95. Reimer C, Deike K, Graf M, et al. Differentiation of pseudoprogression and real progression in glioblastoma using ADC parametric response maps. PLoS One 2017;12(4):e0174620.

96. Gupta A, Young R, Karimi S, et al. Isolated diffusion restriction precedes the development of enhancing tumor in a subset of patients with glioblastoma. AJNR Am J Neuroradiol 2011;32(7):1301–6.

97. Song YS, Choi SH, Park C-K, et al. True progression versus pseudoprogression in the treatment of glioblastomas: a comparison study of normalized cerebral blood volume and apparent diffusion coefficient by histogram analysis. Korean J Radiol 2013;14(4):662–72.

98. Chu HH, Choi SH, Ryoo I, et al. Differentiation of true progression from pseudoprogression in glioblastoma treated with radiation therapy and concomitant temozolomide: comparison study of standard and high-b-value diffusion-weighted imaging. Radiology 2013;269(3):831–40.

99. Nowosielski M, Recheis W, Goebel G, et al. ADC histograms predict response to anti-angiogenic therapy in patients with recurrent high-grade glioma. Neuroradiology 2011;53(4):291–302.

100. Moffat BA, Chenevert TL, Lawrence TS, et al. Functional diffusion map: a noninvasive MRI biomarker for early stratification of clinical brain tumor response. Proc Natl Acad Sci U S A 2005; 102(15):5524–9.

101. Qian X, Tan H, Zhang J, et al. Stratification of pseudoprogression and true progression of glioblastoma multiform based on longitudinal diffusion
tensor imaging without segmentation. Med Phys
2016;43(11):5889–902.
102. Wang S, Martinez-Lage M, Sakai Y, et al. Differentiating tumor progression from pseudoprogression
in patients with glioblastomas using
diffusion tensor imaging and dynamic susceptibility contrast MRI. AJNR Am J Neuroradiol 2016;
37(1):28–36.
103. Agarwal A, Kumar S, Narang J, et al. Morphologic
MRI features, diffusion tensor imaging and radiation dosimetric analysis to differentiate pseudoprogression from early tumor progression.
J Neurooncol 2013;112(3):413–20.
104. Sundgren PC, Fan X, Weybright P, et al. Differentiation of recurrent brain tumor versus radiation
injury using diffusion tensor imaging in patients
with new contrast-enhancing lesions. Magn Reson
Imaging 2006;24(9):1131–42.
105. Soares D, Law M. Magnetic resonance spectroscopy of the brain: review of metabolites and clinical
applications. Clin Radiol 2009;64(1):12–21.
106. Chiang GC, Kovanlikaya I, Choi C, et al. Magnetic
resonance spectroscopy, positron emission tomography and radiogenomics—relevance to glioma.
Front Neurol 2018;9:33.
107. Rees J. Diagnosis and treatment in neuro-
oncology: an oncological perspective. Br J Radiol
2011;84(special_issue_2):S82–9.
108. Pirzkall A, McKnight TR, Graves EE, et al. MR-
spectroscopy guided target delineation for high-
grade gliomas. Int J Radiat Oncol Biol Phys 2001;
50(4):915–28.
109. Graves EE, Nelson SJ, Vigneron DB, et al. Serial
proton MR spectroscopic imaging of recurrent malignant gliomas after gamma knife radiosurgery.
AJNR Am J Neuroradiol 2001;22(4):613–24.
110. Chan AA, Lau A, Pirzkall A, et al. Proton magnetic
resonance spectroscopy imaging in the evaluation
of patients undergoing gamma knife surgery for
Grade IV glioma. J Neurosurg 2004;101(3):467–75.
111. Rock JP, Hearshen D, Scarpace L, et al. Correlations between magnetic resonance spectroscopy
and image-guided histopathology, with special
attention to radiation necrosis. Neurosurgery
2002;51(4):912–20.
112. Lee H, Caparelli E, Li H, et al. Computerized MRS
voxel registration and partial volume effects in single voxel 1H-MRS. Magn Reson Imaging 2013;
31(7):1197–205.
113. Sawlani V, Taylor R, Rowley K, et al. Magnetic resonance spectroscopy for differentiating pseudoprogression from true progression in GBM on concurrent chemoradiotherapy. Neuroradiol J 2012;
25(5):575–86.
114. Kaminaga T, Shirai K. Radiation-induced brain
metabolic changes in the acute and early delayed
phase detected with quantitative proton magnetic
resonance spectroscopy. J Comput Assist Tomogr
2005;29(3):293–7.
115. Andronesi OC, Loebel F, Bogner W, et al. Treatment
response assessment in IDH-mutant glioma patients by noninvasive 3D functional spectroscopic
mapping of 2-hydroxyglutarate. Clin Cancer Res
2016;22(7):1632–41.
116. Choi C, Raisanen JM, Ganji SK, et al. Prospective
longitudinal analysis of 2-hydroxyglutarate magnetic resonance spectroscopy identifies broad
clinical utility for the management of patients
with IDH-mutant glioma. J Clin Oncol 2016;
34(33):4030.
117. Brock C, Young H, O'Reilly S, et al. Early evaluation
of tumour metabolic response using [18 F] fluorodeoxyglucose and positron emission tomography:
a pilot study following the phase II chemotherapy
schedule for temozolomide in recurrent high-
grade gliomas. Br J Cancer 2000;82(3):608.
118. Roelcke U, Von Ammon K, Hausmann O, et al.
Operated low grade astrocytomas: a long term
PET study on the effect of radiotherapy. J Neurol
Neurosurg Psychiatry 1999;66(5):644–7.
119. Hölzer T, Herholz K, Jeske J, et al. FDG-PET as a
prognostic indicator in radiochemotherapy of glioblastoma. J Comput Assist Tomogr 1993;17(5):
681–7.
120. Kim E, Chung S, Haynie T, et al. Differentiation of
residual or recurrent tumors from post-treatment
changes with F-18 FDG PET. Radiographics
1992;12(2):269–79.
121. Wong TZ, Van der Westhuizen GJ, Coleman RE.
Positron emission tomography imaging of brain tumors. Neuroimage Clin 2002;12(4):615–26.
122. Nihashi T, Dahabreh I, Terasawa T. Diagnostic accuracy of PET for recurrent glioma diagnosis: a
meta-analysis. AJNR Am J Neuroradiol 2013;
34(5):944–50.
123. Zikou A, Sioka C, Alexiou GA, et al. Radiation necrosis, pseudoprogression, pseudoresponse, and
tumor recurrence: imaging challenges for the evaluation of treated gliomas. Contrast Media Mol Imaging 2018;2018:6828396.
124. Tripathi M, Sharma R, Varshney R, et al. Comparison of F-18 FDG and C-11 methionine PET/CT for
the evaluation of recurrent primary brain tumors.
Clin Nucl Med 2012;37(2):158–63.
125. Deuschl C, Kirchner J, Poeppel T, et al. 11 C–MET
PET/MRI for detection of recurrent glioma. Eur J
Nucl Med Mol Imaging 2018;45(4):593–601.
126. Galldiks N, Dunkl V, Stoffels G, et al. Diagnosis of
pseudoprogression in patients with glioblastoma
using O-(2-[18 F] fluoroethyl)-L-tyrosine PET. Eur
J Nucl Med Mol Imaging 2015;42(5):685–95.

127. Rachinger W, Goetz C, Pöpperl G, et al. Positron emission tomography with O-(2-[18F] fluoroethyl)-l-tyrosine versus magnetic resonance imaging in the diagnosis of recurrent gliomas. Neurosurgery 2005;57(3):505–11.

128. Kebir S, Khurshid Z, Gaertner FC, et al. Unsupervised consensus cluster analysis of [18F]-fluoroethyl-L-tyrosine positron emission tomography identified textural features for the diagnosis of pseudoprogression in high-grade glioma. Oncotarget 2017;8(5):8294.

129. Mehrkens J, Pöpperl G, Rachinger W, et al. The positive predictive value of O-(2-[18 F] fluoroethyl)-L-tyrosine (FET) PET in the diagnosis of a glioma recurrence after multimodal treatment. J Neurooncol 2008;88(1):27–35.

130. Dunet V, Rossier C, Buck A, et al. Performance of 18F-fluoro-ethyl-tyrosine (18F-FET) PET for the differential diagnosis of primary brain tumor: a systematic review and metaanalysis. J Nucl Med 2012;53(2):207–14.

131. Galldiks N, Langen K-J, Pope WB. From the clinician's point of view: what is the status quo of positron emission tomography in patients with brain tumors? Neuro Oncol 2015;17(11):1434–44.

132. Smith MM, Thompson JE, Castillo M, et al. MR of recurrent high-grade astrocytomas after intralesional immunotherapy. AJNR Am J Neuroradiol 1996;17(6):1065–71.

133. Huang RY, Neagu MR, Reardon DA, et al. Pitfalls in the neuroimaging of glioblastoma in the era of anti-angiogenic and immuno/targeted therapy–detecting illusive disease, defining response. Front Neurol 2015;6:33.

134. Stenberg L, Englund E, Wirestam R, et al. Dynamic susceptibility contrast-enhanced perfusion magnetic resonance (MR) imaging combined with contrast-enhanced MR imaging in the follow-up of immunogene-treated glioblastoma multiforme. Acta Radiol 2006;47(8):852–61.

135. Vrabec M, Van Cauter S, Himmelreich U, et al. MR perfusion and diffusion imaging in the follow-up of recurrent glioblastoma treated with dendritic cell immunotherapy: a pilot study. Neuroradiology 2011;53(10):721–31.

136. Qin L, Li X, Stroiney A, et al. Advanced MRI assessment to predict benefit of anti-programmed cell death 1 protein immunotherapy response in patients with recurrent glioblastoma. Neuroradiology 2017;59(2):135–45.

137. Floeth F, Wittsack H-J, Engelbrecht V, et al. Comparative follow-up of enhancement phenomena with MRI and proton MR spectroscopic imaging after intralesional immunotherapy in glioblastoma. Zentralbl Neurochir 2002;63(01):23–8.

138. Pellegatta S, Eoli M, Frigerio S, et al. The natural killer cell response and tumor debulking are associated with prolonged survival in recurrent glioblastoma patients receiving dendritic cells loaded with autologous tumor lysates. Oncoimmunology 2013;2(3):e23401.

139. Wang N, Jain RK, Batchelor TT. New directions in anti-angiogenic therapy for glioblastoma. Neurotherapeutics 2017;14(2):321–32.

140. Jain RK, Di Tomaso E, Duda DG, et al. Angiogenesis in brain tumours. Nat Rev Neurosci 2007; 8(8):610.

141. Batchelor TT, Sorensen AG, di Tomaso E, et al. AZD2171, a pan-VEGF receptor tyrosine kinase inhibitor, normalizes tumor vasculature and alleviates edema in glioblastoma patients. Cancer Cell 2007; 11(1):83–95.

142. Friedman HS, Prados MD, Wen PY, et al. Bevacizumab alone and in combination with irinotecan in recurrent glioblastoma. J Clin Oncol 2009;27(28): 4733–40.

143. Norden A, Young G, Setayesh K, et al. Bevacizumab for recurrent malignant gliomas. Efficacy, toxicity, and patterns of recurrence. Neurology 2008;70(10):779–87.

144. Boxerman JL, Zhang Z, Safriel Y, et al. Prognostic value of contrast enhancement and FLAIR for survival in newly diagnosed glioblastoma treated with and without bevacizumab: results from ACRIN 6686. Neuro Oncol 2018;20(10):1400–10.

145. Stadlbauer A, Pichler P, Karl M, et al. Quantification of serial changes in cerebral blood volume and metabolism in patients with recurrent glioblastoma undergoing antiangiogenic therapy. Eur J Radiol 2015;84(6):1128–36.

146. Sorensen AG, Emblem KE, Polaskova P, et al. Increased survival of glioblastoma patients who respond to antiangiogenic therapy with elevated blood perfusion. Cancer Res 2012;72(2):402–7.

147. Hilario A, Sepulveda J, Hernandez-Lain A, et al. Leakage decrease detected by dynamic susceptibility-weighted contrast-enhanced perfusion MRI predicts survival in recurrent glioblastoma treated with bevacizumab. Clin Transl Oncol 2017; 19(1):51–7.

148. Auer TA, Breit H-C, Marini F, et al. Evaluation of the apparent diffusion coefficient in patients with recurrent glioblastoma under treatment with bevacizumab with radiographic pseudoresponse. J Neuroradiol 2019;46(1):36–43.

149. Ellingson BM, Gerstner ER, Smits M, et al. Diffusion MRI phenotypes predict overall survival benefit from anti-VEGF monotherapy in recurrent glioblastoma: converging evidence from phase II trials. Clin Cancer Res 2017;23(19):5745–56.

150. Galldiks N, Rapp M, Stoffels G, et al. Earlier diagnosis of progressive disease during bevacizumab treatment using O-(2-18F-fluoroethyl)-L-tyrosine positron emission tomography in comparison with

magnetic resonance imaging. Mol Imaging 2013; 12(5):273–6.

151. Schwarzenberg J, Czernin J, Cloughesy TF, et al. Treatment response evaluation using 18F-FDOPA PET in patients with recurrent malignant glioma on bevacizumab therapy. Clin Cancer Res 2014; 20(13):3550–9.

152. Alexiou GA, Zikou A, Tsiouris S, et al. Comparison of diffusion tensor, dynamic susceptibility contrast MRI and 99mTc-Tetrofosmin brain SPECT for the detection of recurrent high-grade glioma. Magn Reson Imaging 2014;32(7):854–9.

153. Gasparetto EL, Pawlak MA, Patel SH, et al. Post-treatment recurrence of malignant brain neoplasm: accuracy of relative cerebral blood volume fraction in discriminating low from high malignant histologic volume fraction. Radiology 2009;250(3):887–96.

154. Narang J, Jain R, Arbab AS, et al. Differentiating treatment-induced necrosis from recurrent/progressive brain tumor using nonmodel-based semiquantitative indices derived from dynamic contrast-enhanced T1-weighted MR perfusion. Neuro Oncol 2011;13(9):1037–46.

155. Rahmathulla G, Marko NF, Weil RJ. Cerebral radiation necrosis: a review of the pathobiology, diagnosis and management considerations. J Clin Neurosci 2013;20(4):485–502.

156. Marks JE, Baglan RJ, Prassad SC, et al. Cerebral radionecrosis: incidence and risk in relation to dose, time, fractionation and volume. Int J Radiat Oncol Biol Phys 1981;7(2):243–52.

157. Acharya S, Robinson CG, Michalski JM, et al. Association of 1p/19q codeletion and radiation necrosis in adult cranial gliomas after proton or photon therapy. Int J Radiat Oncol Biol Phys 2018;101(2): 334–43.

158. Kumar AJ, Leeds NE, Fuller GN, et al. Malignant gliomas: MR imaging spectrum of radiation therapy-and chemotherapy-induced necrosis of the brain after treatment. Radiology 2000;217(2): 377–84.

159. Aiken AH, Chang SM, Larson D, et al. Longitudinal magnetic resonance imaging features of glioblastoma multiforme treated with radiotherapy with or without brachytherapy. Int J Radiat Oncol Biol Phys 2008;72(5):1340–6.

160. Ryken TC, Aygun N, Morris J, et al. The role of imaging in the management of progressive glioblastoma. J Neurooncol 2014;118(3):435–60.

161. Al Sayyari A, Buckley R, McHenery C, et al. Distinguishing recurrent primary brain tumor from radiation injury: a preliminary study using a susceptibility-weighted MR imaging– guided apparent diffusion coefficient analysis strategy. AJNR Am J Neuroradiol 2010;31(6):1049–54.

162. Ringelstein A, Turowski B, Gizewski E, et al. Evaluation of ADC mapping as an early predictor for

tumor response to chemotherapy in recurrent glioma treated with bevacizumab/irinotecan: proof of principle. RoFo 2010;182(10):868–72.

163. Pica A, Hauf M, Slotboom J, et al. P. 074* dynamic susceptibility contrast perfusion MRI in differentiating radiation necrosis from tumor recurrence in high-grade gliomas. Neuro Oncol 2012;14(suppl_ 3):iii1–94.

164. Barajas RF Jr, Chang JS, Segal MR, et al. Differentiation of recurrent glioblastoma multiforme from radiation necrosis after external beam radiation therapy with dynamic susceptibility-weighted contrast-enhanced perfusion MR imaging. Radiology 2009;253(2):486–96.

165. Larsen VA, Simonsen HJ, Law I, et al. Evaluation of dynamic contrast-enhanced T1-weighted perfusion MRI in the differentiation of tumor recurrence from radiation necrosis. Neuroradiology 2013; 55(3):361–9.

166. Ozsunar Y, Mullins ME, Kwong K, et al. Glioma recurrence versus radiation necrosis? A pilot comparison of arterial spin-labeled, dynamic susceptibility contrast enhanced MRI, and FDG-PET imaging. Acad Radiol 2010;17(3):282–90.

167. Srinivasan R, Phillips JJ, VandenBerg SR, et al. Ex vivo MR spectroscopic measure differentiates tumor from treatment effects in GBM. Neuro Oncol 2010;12(11):1152–61.

168. Weybright P, Sundgren PC, Maly P, et al. Differentiation between brain tumor recurrence and radiation injury using MR spectroscopy. AJR Am J Roentgenol 2005;185(6):1471–6.

169. Rabinov JD, Lee PL, Barker FG, et al. In vivo 3-T MR spectroscopy in the distinction of recurrent glioma versus radiation effects: initial experience. Radiology 2002;225(3):871–9.

170. Wald LL, Nelson SJ, Day MR, et al. Serial proton magnetic resonance spectroscopy imaging of glioblastoma multiforme after brachytherapy. J Neurosurg 1997;87(4):525–34.

171. Enslow MS, Zollinger LV, Morton KA, et al. Comparison of F-18 fluorodeoxyglucose and F-18 fluorothymidine positron emission tomography in differentiating radiation necrosis from recurrent glioma. Clin Nucl Med 2012;37(9):854.

172. Rollin N, Guyotat J, Streichenberger N, et al. Clinical relevance of diffusion and perfusion magnetic resonance imaging in assessing intra-axial brain tumors. Neuroradiology 2006;48(3): 150–9.

173. Kim YH, Oh SW, Lim YJ, et al. Differentiating radiation necrosis from tumor recurrence in high-grade gliomas: assessing the efficacy of 18F-FDG PET, 11C-methionine PET and perfusion MRI. Clin Neurol Neurosurg 2010;112(9):758–65.

174. Chernov M, Hayashi M, Izawa M, et al. Differentiation of the radiation-induced necrosis and tumor

recurrence after gamma knife radiosurgery for brain metastases: importance of multi-voxel proton MRS. Minim Invasive Neurosurg 2005;48(04): 228–34.

175. Zhang H, Ma L, Wang Q, et al. Role of magnetic resonance spectroscopy for the differentiation of recurrent glioma from radiation necrosis: a systematic review and meta-analysis. Eur J Radiol 2014; 83(12):2181–9.

176. Pötzi C, Becherer A, Marosi C, et al. [11C] methionine and [18F] fluorodeoxyglucose PET in the follow-up of glioblastoma multiforme. J Neurooncol 2007;84(3):305.

177. Hollingworth W, Medina L, Lenkinski R, et al. A systematic literature review of magnetic resonance spectroscopy for the characterization of brain tumors. AJNR Am J Neuroradiol 2006;27(7): 1404–11.

Adult Primary Brain Neoplasm, Including 2016 World Health Organization Classification

Kevin Yuqi Wang, MD[a], Melissa M. Chen, MD[b], Christie M. Malayil Lincoln, MD[a],*

KEYWORDS

• WHO • Central nervous system • MR imaging • Adult primary neoplasm

KEY POINTS

• The 2016 update to the fourth edition of the World Health Organization central nervous system (CNS) tumor classification scheme represents a fundamental change in the manner in which tumors are classified and for the first time incorporates molecular parameters in addition to traditional microscopic features into the updated classification scheme.
• The most impactful changes involve classification of diffuse gliomas, with the incorporation of genetically defined features.
• Molecular markers of the genetically defined tumors are not only of diagnostic significance but also of prognostic value; examples include isocitrate dehydrogenase mutations and 1p/19q codeletions in astrocytomas and oligodendrogliomas, respectively.
• Imaging remains a mainstay modality in the diagnosis and management of adult primary CNS tumors, and familiarity with the new scheme is crucial for neuroradiologists to convey meaningful information to their referring colleagues.

INTRODUCTION

Updates in the 2016 World Health Organization Central Nervous System Tumor Classification

Primary central nervous system (CNS) tumors are the seventh most common adult neoplasm,[1] with an overall incidence rate of 23 cases per 100,000 people in the United States.[2] The most widely accepted classification scheme is based on the World Health Organization (WHO) classification of tumors of the CNS, currently in its fourth edition. For nearly the past century, the classification of CNS tumors was traditionally based on microscopic features, with the assumption that tumors could be classified according to histologic similarities based on the cells of origin (eg, astrocytomas originating from astrocytes or oligodendrogliomas originating from oligodendrocytes) and further subclassified based on their degree of cellular differentiation.[3] The past 2 decades of genetic and epigenetic research, however, have clarified the basis of tumorigenesis in a manner that has fundamentally altered the classification system. In the 2016 WHO classification, an update to the fourth edition represents a major paradigm shift in the manner in which CNS tumors are classified, for the first time integrating molecular parameters (genotypic) into the traditional microscopic features (phenotypic).[4]

This article was previously published in *Radiology Clinics of North America*, Volume 57, Number 6, Pages 1147-1162.

[a] Department of Radiology, Baylor College of Medicine, One Baylor Plaza, MS360, Houston, TX 77030, USA;
[b] Department of Diagnostic Radiology, Division of Diagnostic Imaging, The University of Texas MD Anderson Cancer Center, 1400 Pressler Street, Unit 1482, Houston, TX 77030, USA
* Corresponding author. One Baylor Plaza, MS360, Houston, TX 77030.
E-mail address: Christie.Lincoln@bcm.edu

Neuroimag Clin N Am 31 (2021) 121–138
https://doi.org/10.1016/j.nic.2020.09.011

The implications of this updated classification are both broad and deep. For example, prognoses of certain tumors often correlate more strongly with molecular markers than with histologic grade (eg, isocitrate dehydrogenase [IDH] mutation status). The presence of molecular markers adds a level of objectivity and reproducibility conspicuously missing in a diagnostic process solely dependent on microscopic observation (eg, oligodendroglioma).[3] Reconciling discordance between genotypic and phenotypic parameters is now an issue. For example, a glioma that histologically and phenotypically appears astrocytic may possess a 1p/19q codeletion, a genotypic parameter that is almost always seen in oligodendrogliomas. Conversely, a tumor that histologically resembles oligodendroglioma may possess ATRX and TP53 mutations with an intact 1p and 19q, which are molecular signatures genotypically consistent with astrocytomas. Therefore, familiarity with the new classification scheme is critical for neuroradiologists to convey meaningful information for optimal collaborative disease management by radiation oncologists, neuropathologists, neuro-oncologists, and neurosurgeons.

Classification Considerations: Layered Diagnosis, Not Otherwise Specified, Not Elsewhere Classified

The concept of a layered diagnosis was introduced to assist in systematically diagnosing CNS tumors, incorporating both genotypic and phenotypic parameters into the diagnosis.[4,5] Layer 1 represents the integrated diagnosis, whereby a unifying summation of the molecular and microscopic data most accurately represents the diagnostic entity and can be generated only if information from all other layers are present. Layer 2 represents the histologic classification (eg, oligodendroglioma). Layer 3 presents the WHO grade (eg, WHO grade III). Layer 4 represents the molecular parameters (eg, 1p/19q codeletion). A layer 2 and 3 diagnosis can be made when no molecular data are available and is used to convey that a full, integrated layer 1 diagnosis is not possible.

The suffix not otherwise specified (NOS) is a designation in the 2016 WHO classification that denotes that the necessary molecular assays were unavailable or not performed at the facility to provide a layer 4 diagnosis for entities that may qualify for an integrated layer 1 diagnosis (eg, oligodendrogliomas, astrocytomas, or embryonal tumors). Therefore, the suffix conveys through the pathology report that the case has not been worked up to the necessary extent for a full, integrated layer 1 diagnosis. In contrast, the suffix, not elsewhere classified (NEC), is a designation used when molecular data analyses are performed and available, but the histologic (layer 2 and 3) and molecular (layer 4) data altogether are conflicting, therefore preventing a consensus diagnosis. It also may be used for increasingly well-described genetically defined entities for which there is no official recognition by the WHO classification scheme. This suffix is not yet codified in the 2016 WHO classification but likely will be utilized in the upcoming fifth edition.[6] For example, the NEC designation can be used in cases of histologically classic oligodendroglioma with an IDH-type molecular marker or histologically classic diffuse astrocytoma with molecular features of glioblastoma. NEC also can be used with new molecular entities, such as glioblastoma, *FGFR3-TACC3* fusion, which is resistant to conventional chemoradiation. It becomes important for the neuropathologist to identify these gliomas for inclusion in targeted therapeutic trials.[7]

Goals and Objectives

Although a comprehensive review of adult primary brain neoplasms based on the 2016 WHO classification is outside the scope of this article, the goal is to impart the readership with a working knowledge of the typical MR imaging findings of commonly encountered adult primary brain neoplasms and the relevant changes in 2016 WHO classification.

IMAGING TECHNIQUE AND CONSIDERATIONS

Imaging plays a major role as it represents the modern-day gross specimen. A differential diagnosis in order of probability can be formulated by scrutinizing all sources of information from a patient's clinical and demographic features (age, gender, and presenting symptoms/signs) to imaging findings: anatomic location, borders, and tissue characteristics of the lesion as well as the presence and pattern of contrast enhancement. A routine brain MR image offers conventional sequences used to evaluate brain tumors, including precontrast and postcontrast T1-weighted imaging (T1WI), T2-weighted imaging (T2WI), T2-weighted fluid-attenuated inversion recovery (FLAIR), diffusion-weighted imaging (DWI), and either gradient-recalled echo (GRE) or susceptibility-weighted imaging (SWI). Small field-of-view, thin-slice sagittal T2WI and sagittal postcontrast T1WI provide the best diagnostic value for tackling pineal region tumors. High-resolution T2WI, constructive interference in steady state, or fast imaging employing steady-state acquisition sequences of the cerebellopontine angle and internal auditory canal can be used to evaluate vestibular schwannomas. Small field-of-view, thin-slice precontrast and postcontrast images as well as postcontrast dynamic images are helpful when assessing sellar region neoplasms. Unless explicitly stated as otherwise, imaging findings discussed within this article are based on MR imaging.

PATHOLOGY AND IMAGING
Diffusely Infiltrating Gliomas

Gliomas represent a diverse and heterogeneous group of tumors. Based on the traditional phenotypic classification scheme, gliomas were thought to arise from a glial cell of origin. Therefore, subtypes of glial cells, such as astrocytes and oligodendrocytes, give rise to specific types of glioma, astrocytoma and oligodendroglioma, respectively.[1] Gliomas can be relatively circumscribed with a tendency toward benignity (eg, pleomorphic xanthoastrocytoma, pilocytic astrocytoma, and subependymal giant cell astrocytoma) or diffusely infiltrating with tendency toward malignancy (eg, diffuse astrocytoma and oligodendroglioma). Previously, in the 2007 WHO classification, all astrocytic tumors were grouped together. Due to differences in growth pattern and behavior between circumscribed and diffusely infiltrating gliomas, all diffusely infiltrating gliomas are now amassed into 1 category regardless of histologic subtype (eg, astrocytic or oligodendroglial).[4] Based on the 2016 WHO classification, diffusely infiltrating gliomas are composed of diffusely infiltrating astrocytomas, glioblastomas, and oligodendrogliomas.

Diffuse and anaplastic astrocytoma

After histologic confirmation and grading of diffusely infiltrating astrocytoms, including WHO grade II diffuse astrocytomas (not to be confused with the general term, diffusely infiltrating astrocytomas) and WHO grade III anaplastic astrocytomas (grade III), these tumors are further stratified by IDH mutations. Approximately 90% of grades II and III diffusely infiltrating astrocytomas are IDH-mutants.[1] Diffuse astrocytoma IDH–wild-type is such an uncommon diagnosis that reevaluation of an alternative diagnosis is often required.[4] Anaplastic astrocytoma IDH–wild-type also is uncommon, with most tumors sharing genetic features with those of glioblastoma IDH–wild-type.[4] Several recent studies have suggest minimal prognostic difference between grade II and grade III IDH-mutant astrocytomas[4] and further suggest that IDH status serves as a more accurate prognostic marker (IDH-mutant more favorable than IDH–wild-type)

than WHO grading. At this time, however, the WHO grading scheme along with IDH status is retained; amendments are likely to occur in the next revision.[3]

On imaging, diffusely infiltrating astrocytomas are T2/FLAIR hyperintense masses that frequently arise from the cerebral hemispheres, with predilection for the frontal lobes. Despite their infiltrating growth pattern, they appear relatively circumscribed on imaging, tend to involve the underlying white matter, and are associated with characteristic cortical infiltration and gyral expansion. Both diffuse and anaplastic astrocytomas typically do not restrict on DWI and do not enhance with contrast. Enhancement is variably present in anaplastic astrocytomas (**Figs. 1** and **2**). Ultimately, no distinctive imaging features reliably distinguish astrocytomas by WHO grade and IDH status.

Glioblastoma

Glioblastoma is a grade IV diffusely infiltrating astrocytoma that is also further stratified by IDH mutation status. Glioblastoma IDH–wild-type type arises de novo (clinically defined as primary glioblastoma), whereas glioblastoma IDH-mutant arises from a lower-grade IDH-mutant diffusely infiltrating astrocytoma (clinically defined as secondary glioblastoma).[8] Unlike astrocytoma, approximately 90% to 95% of glioblastomas are IDH–wild-type, tend to occur in patients greater than 55 years old, and portend a worse prognosis compared with IDH-mutants.[1,8] Despite arising de novo, glioblastoma IDH–wild-type shares other genetic alterations (eg, *TERT* promoter, *EGFR* amplification, and *PTEN* mutations) as well as clinical features with diffusely infiltrating astrocytoma IDH–wild-type,[1,4] perhaps reflecting a spectrum of the same entity.

The term, *multifocal, glioblastoma*, often is used when referring to multiple, seemingly separate foci of tumor that are connected by spread of disease via white matter tracts or cerebrospinal fluid. On the other hand, the term, *multicentric glioblastoma*, often is used when there is no obvious imaging finding demonstrating a connection among separate tumor foci. Glioblastoma IDH–wild-type tumors classically demonstrate a thick, irregular rind of enhancing tumor, which histologically correlates with vascular proliferation. Centrally, a nonenhancing necrotic core typically preferentially involves the subcortical and deep white matter (**Fig. 3**) on postcontrast T1WI. T2/FLAIR sequences demonstrate a poorly marginated, heterogeneously hyperintense mass with mass effect and extensive vasogenic edema. Tumor invariably extends beyond the regions of

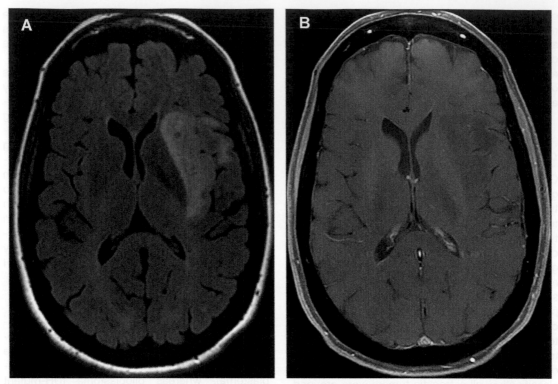

Fig. 1. Anaplastic astrocytoma, IDH-mutant on axial FLAIR and T1 postcontrast images manifests as a large cortical and subcortical nonenhancing area (*B*) of increasing signal (*A*) in the left lateral putamen, extreme capsule, insular cortex, and frontal operculum.

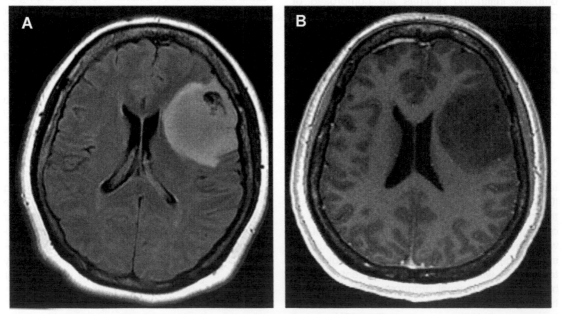

Fig. 2. A patient with diffuse astrocytoma, IDH-mutant with a larger nonenhancing area (*D*) of increased signal (*A*) in the left middle and inferior frontal gyri and operculum. Despite the size of the lesions in the index case, there is no subfalcine herniation or effacement of the lateral ventricles.

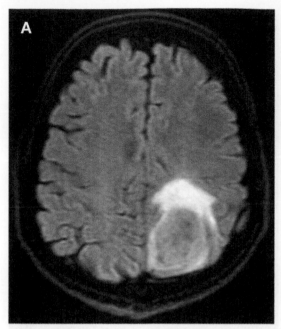
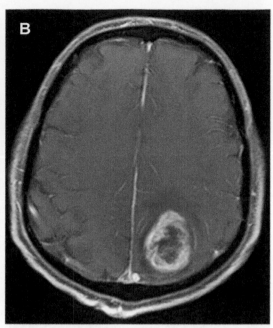

Fig. 3. Glioblastoma, IDH–wild-type exhibits a thick irregular ring of contrast enhancement (*B*) and central necrotic core with extensive vasogenic edema (*A*) in the left parietal lobe.

enhancement, even beyond the extent of visible peritumoral edema, frequently along white matter tracts; this is referred to as microscopic invasion. The moniker, butterfly glioma, has been used when symmetric corpus callosum involvement is present. Nonenhancing tumor and vasogenic edema are virtually indistinguishable radiologically. Tumor heterogeneity is often due to a combination of necrosis and intratumoral hemorrhage; the latter is common and easily elucidated on GRE or SWI. Calcification and restricted diffusion are rare.

In contrast to astrocytomas, certain imaging findings may help distinguish glioblastoma IDH-mutants from IDH–wild-type. Glioblastoma IDH-mutants preferentially involve the frontal lobes[4] and commonly have regions of nonenhancing tumor, not including the admixture of peritumoral edema/tumor.[1] The thick enhancing rind, intratumoral hemorrhage, and large centrally necrotic components, which are classic features of glioblastoma IDH–wild-type, are infrequent features in glioblastoma IDH-mutants (**Fig. 4**).

Oligodendroglioma

Oligodendroglioma (WHO grade II) and anaplastic oligodendroglioma (WHO grade III) share the same IDH gene family mutation as diffusely infiltrating astrocytomas. Oligodendrogliomas often are distinguished from astrocytomas by the presence of an additional 1p/19q codeletion. The less frequently encountered histologically classic oligodendroglioma with IDH–wild-type is given the diagnosis oligodendroglioma, NOS, after exclusion of other possible entities. In addition to its diagnostic value, the presence of a 1p/19q codeletion is prognostically significant in diffuse gliomas. Those with the codeletion receiving radiation followed by procarbazine, lomustine, and vincristine chemotherapy demonstrate significantly higher survival rates compared with those without the codeletion.[9–11] In contrast, similar to astrocytomas, the prognostic value of grading remains an issue, because several studies have failed to identify a difference in survival by WHO grade after IDH mutation status stratification.[12–14] Amendments to this histology-driven grading scheme may occur in the upcoming revision of the WHO classification scheme.[5]

Oligoastrocytomas were previously diagnosed based on the histologic admixture of both astrocytic and oligodendrolglial components; however, due to high interobserver variability, this criterion is strongly discouraged in the 2016 WHO classification. The vast majority of diffuse gliomas with histologic features of both astrocytic and oligodendroglial components can now be confidently classified as purely astrocytoma or oligodendroglioma based on genetic testing.[4]

On imaging, oligodendrogliomas occur predominantly supratentorially, with preference for the frontal lobes (50%–65%).[1] These tumors are

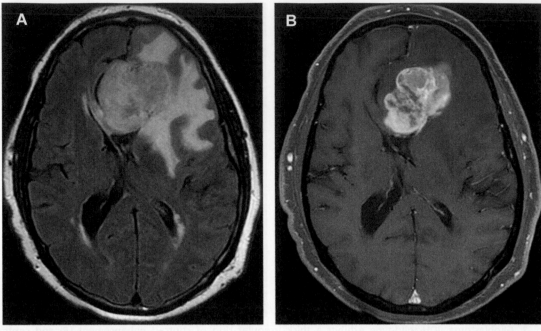

Fig. 4. Glioblastoma, IDH-mutant involves the left frontal lobe with more heterogeneous and solid areas of enhancement (*B*) and regions where there is nonenhancing tumor and vasogenic edema (*A*) in the white matter of the left frontal lobe and subinsular and extreme capsule region.

relatively well defined, cortically based T2/FLAIR hyperintense masses with associated gyral expansion, occasional remodeling of the overlying calvarium, and frequent intratumoral coarse calcifications (**Fig. 5**). Preoperative calcification was found significantly predictive of the 1p/19q codeletion.[15] Peritumoral edema, hemorrhage, and necrosis are less common features. Similar to diffusely infiltrating astrocytomas, enhancement is inconsistent, with approximately 50% of cases manifesting some degree of enhancement, which is also unreliable in distinguishing grade II from grade III tumors.[1]

Diffuse midline glioma, H3 K27M-mutant

Diffuse midline gliomas, H3 K27M-mutant, are a new grade IV entity in the 2016 WHO classification. Although these tumors are classically seen in pediatric patients, recent studies demonstrate that they are not infrequently encountered in the adult population.[16,17] A recent case series of such tumors in adults reported the age range from ages 28 years to 81 years, with a median age of 52 years. Prognosis in the adult population is poor, similar to that in the pediatric population, with mean survival of 9.3 months.[16]

Typically found in the thalamus, pons, or hypothalamus, these tumors present as expansile T2/FLAIR hyperintense masses with variable enhancement (**Fig. 6**). Interestingly, 2 of the 4

criteria for pathologic diagnosis of this tumor are based on its imaging appearance. The tumors must appear diffuse and midline in addition to supporting the histologic diagnosis of glioma with the genetic mutation of H3 K27M.[18] Leptomeningeal dissemination has been reported.[16]

Ependymal Tumors

Ependymal tumors are a heterogeneous group of tumors that share histopathologic similarities despite arising from various anatomic sites across the neuroaxis.[1] The genetics and tumorigenesis of ependymomas are less well elucidated than in diffuse gliomas. Several studies have demonstrated limited value in the currently established histology-based classification and grading system.[19] Nevertheless, a few revisions were made in the 2016 WHO classification, because the presence of molecular markers to identify these subtypes is still forthcoming in most instances.[5,20,21] The exception is the ependymoma, *RELA* fusion-positive subtype, which comprises a majority of pediatric supratentorial tumors.[4,22] Moreover, with exception of myxopapillary ependymomas and subependymomas, a majority of ependymal tumors are seen in the pediatric population.

Subependymoma

Subependymomas are rare, slow-growing, WHO grade I tumors often found incidentally on imaging

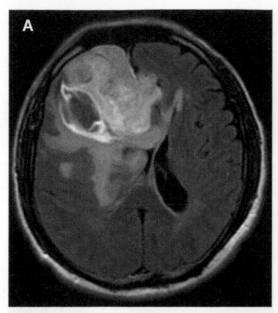
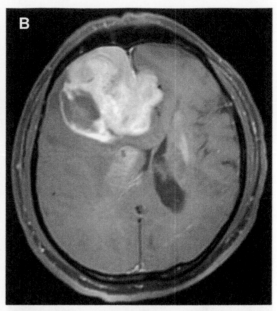

Fig. 5. Anaplastic oligodendroglioma, IDH-mutant, and 1p/19q-codeleted with well circumscribed, cortical-based, right frontal FLAIR hyperintense (A) and nearly homogenously enhancing tumor (B) with a small nonenhancing component and extensive vasogenic edema resulting in subfalcine herniation and partial effacement of the lateral ventricles. On CT (not shown), there was associated remodeling of the inner table of the right frontal calvarium and coarse calcifications within the tumor.

or autopsy in middle-aged to older adults.[1] If patients are symptomatic, it is usually secondary to obstructive hydrocephalus.

On imaging, approximately half of cases are found at the frontal horns of the lateral ventricles in close association with the septum pellucidum. The second most common location is in the fourth ventricle. They are well circumscribed, heterogeneously T2/FLAIR hyperintense masses that may expand the ventricle but otherwise demonstrate minimal mass effect (Fig. 7). When large, they may cause obstructive hydrocephalus. Other

common imaging features include calcification and intratumoral cysts. These tumors show variable enhancement and rarely demonstrate restricted diffusion or hemorrhage.

Neuronal and Glioneuronal Tumors

Neuronal and mixed glioneuronal tumors are those that contain purely neurocytic or an admixture of neurocytic and glial elements, respectively. Glioneuronal tumors often are associated with clinical presentation of seizures, are lower in incidence

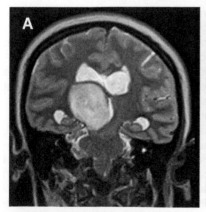
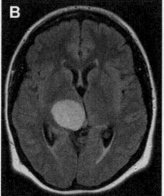
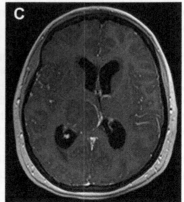

Fig. 6. A right thalamic diffuse midline glioma illustrates increased T2 (A) and FLAIR signal (B) and does not enhance (C). Despite the large size, there is no vasogenic edema; however, there is regional mass effect.

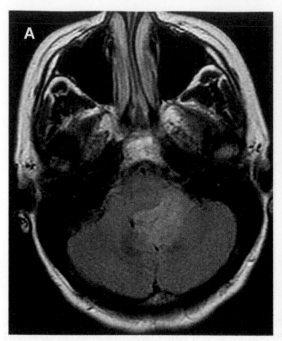
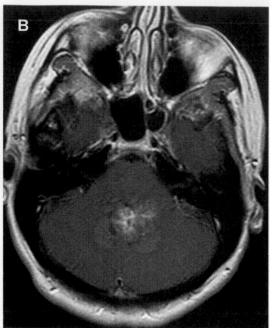

Fig. 7. A subependymoma expands the fourth ventricle and is a FLAIR hyperintense mass (*A*) with nonspecific, heterogeneous enhancement (*B*).

than pure gliomas, and are associated with a better prognosis.[1] A majority of these neoplasms are designated WHO grade I.

Ganglioglioma and anaplastic ganglioglioma

Gangliogliomas are tumors histologically composed of a mix of neoplastic ganglion and glial elements. They are the most common glioneuronal tumor and the majority occur in children and young adults. As with many glioneuronal tumors, medically-refractory epilepsy is the typical presentation. The majority are benign, very indolent tumors and are, therefore, designated WHO grade I. Anaplastic gangliogliomas are relatively more rare, comprising only 8% to 10% of all gangliogliomas.[1] They are aggressive WHO grade III tumors; often, the glial component demonstrates malignant features histologically.[1]

On imaging, gangliogliomas arise most frequently in the temporal lobes as well defined, cortically based T2/FLAIR hyperintense lesions with solid and cystic components (Fig. 8). An enhancing mural nodule is typically seen arising from the cystic component of the tumor. Imaging features cannot reliably distinguish between benign and anaplastic gangliogliomas, although the latter may demonstrate more ill-defined margins and occur in more atypical locations.[1]

Gangliocytoma

Unlike gangliogliomas, gangliocytomas are benign neoplasms comprised exclusively of ganglion cells without glial elements, designated as WHO grade I. Similar to gangliogliomas, however, they occur frequently in children and young adults, often presenting with medically refractory epilepsy.

Imaging findings of gangliocytomas are indistinguishable from those of gangliogliomas. The typical location and imaging appearance is a cortically based T2/FLAIR hyperintense solid and cystic mass most frequently in the temporal lobe (Fig. 9). The solid components variably demonstrate intense homogeneous enhancement. Calcification within the solid components may be seen in approximately one-third of cases.[1]

Dysplastic cerebellar gangliocytoma

Also known as Lhermitte-Duclos disease, dysplastic cerebellar gangliocytoma is a slow-growing, infratentorial, benign, WHO grade I lesion of either neoplastic or hamartomatous nature. A majority of lesions are sporadic although may be seen in association with an autosomal-dominant phakomatosis, known as Cowden syndrome.[1]

As the name suggests, the lesion typically appears as a relatively well-defined, unilateral, expansile mass involving and replacing the cerebellar hemisphere and/or vermis. Mass effect and effacement of the fourth ventricle are common and can result in obstructive hydrocephalus. T2/FLAIR imaging demonstrates a characteristic gyriform and striated pattern of the lesion, reflecting the alternating intensities of the expanded and

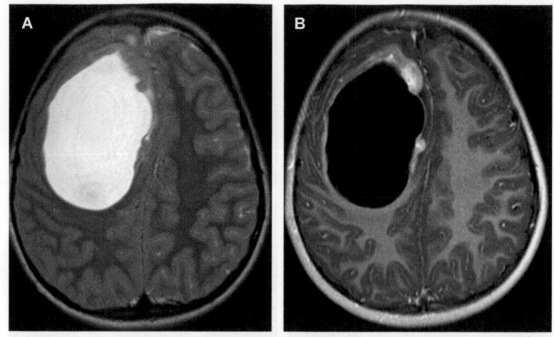

Fig. 8. A patient with right frontal cortical-based ganglioglioma that has a large FLAIR hyperintense cystic component (*A*), with solid peripheral enhancing mural nodules in the anterior and medial wall of the cyst (*B*).

thickened cerebellar folia (**Fig. 10**). The tumor may restrict on DWI, perhaps reflecting its increased cellularity. Although enhancement is typically absent, enhancing vessels can be seen traversing the lesion and can be confirmed on T2WI, GRE, or SWI as signal void structures related to flow in the vasculature.

Rosette-forming glioneuronal tumor
Rosette-forming glioneuronal tumors are benign, slow-growing tumors of WHO grade I. The

attribute, "of the fourth ventricle," has been removed from its name in the 2016 WHO classification, because it also occasionally may arise from the cerebellar vermis, cerebellar hemisphere, and pineal region, among other locations.[5] Rosette-forming glioneuronal tumors typically occur in young adults, with peak incidence in the third decade.[23]

Imaging typically demonstrates a markedly heterogeneous cystic and solid mass, mostly commonly located midline within the fourth

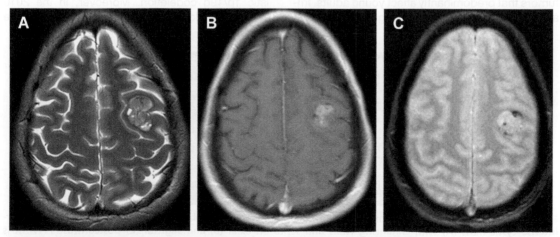

Fig. 9. A left frontal cortically based gangliocytoma with solid and cystic T2 areas (*A*), intense enhancement of the solid component (*B*), and areas of coarse calcification seen on gradient imaging (*C*).

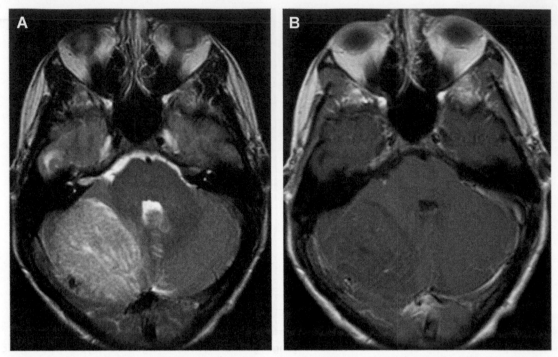

Fig. 10. An index case of right dysplastic cerebellar gangliocytoma that is nonenhancing (*B*), expansile, well defined, striated and gyriform pattern and replaces the entire right cerebellum (*A*). There is partial effacement of the fourth ventricle, and there are some enhancing vessels in the substance of this WHO grade I lesion (*B*).

ventricle or cerebellar vermis with variable presence of intratumoral hemorrhage, fluid-fluid levels, and calcification (**Fig. 11**). Heterogeneous and patchy enhancement is typical; CSF dissemination may occur.

Papillary glioneuronal tumor

Previously considered a ganglioglioma subtype, papillary glioneuronal tumors are now distinctly classified. They are slow-growing, WHO grade I tumors that predominantly affect young adults. Imaging findings are indistinguishable from

gangliogliomas and include a well-defined mixed cystic and solid mass, most frequently arising from the temporal lobes (**Fig. 12**).

Central neurocytoma

Central neurocytomas are benign, WHO grade II, intraventricular tumors with purely neurocytic elements, therefore originally thought to be a subtype of oligodendrogliomas. These tumors lack glial components, however, as well as the characteristic 1p/19q codeletion. Moreover, in the 2016 WHO classification, they are defined by the

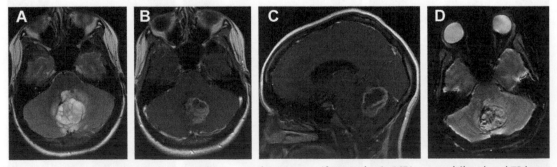

Fig. 11. A patient with Rosette-forming glioneuronal tumor manifests on brain MRI as a multiloculated T2 hyperintense cystic mass (*A*) with enhancing walls and septa on axial (*B*) and sagittal (*C*) postcontrast T1WI. It is centered in the posterior fourth ventricle and vermis, and there is also the presence of intratumoral hemorrhage, as shown on SWI (*D*).

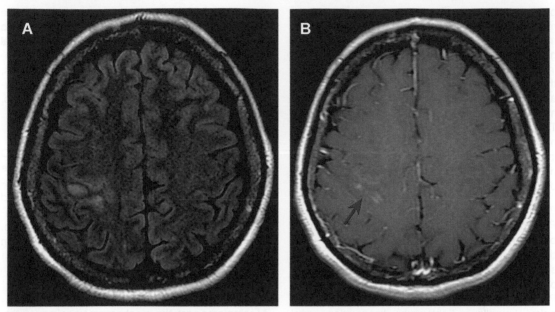

Fig. 12. A papillary glioneuronal tumor shows well circumscribed, cortical-based right parietal lobe FLAIR signal change (*A*) and wispy punctate and linear enhancement (*red arrow* [*B*]).

absence of IDH mutations,[5] further distinguishing them from oligodendrogliomas. They represent the most common primary intraventricular neoplasm of young to middle-aged adults.[1] Although slow-growing, central neurocytomas may result in sudden obstructive hydrocephalus due to their location.

On imaging, a well-defined heterogeneous, bubbly, T2/FLAIR hyperintense mass typically arises from in the body of the lateral ventricle near the foramen of Monro, attached to the septum pellucidum[1] (**Fig. 13**). Calcification, intratumoral cysts, vascular flow-related signal void, and marked heterogeneous enhancement are common.

Pineal Gland Tumors

The approach to pineal gland tumors can be simplified into 2 broad categories: pineal

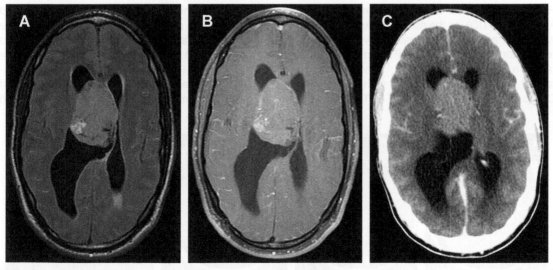

Fig. 13. A FLAIR hyperintense (*A*) and mildly enhancing (*B*) central neurocytoma is demonstrated in the body of the right lateral ventricle with bowing the septum pellucidum to the left and obstructive hydrocephalus. The axial head CT with contrast shows mild enhancement of the large right lateral ventricle lesion and obstructive hydrocephalus (*C*).

parenchymal and germ cell tumors. Germ cell tumors are the most common group of pineal tumors, predominantly seen in the pediatric age group. Because they occupy a separate category in the WHO classification, they are described in the following section. Pineal parenchymal tumors arise from pinealocytes and comprise approximately 15% to 30% of all pineal gland tumors.[1] Though not the focus of this article, many other neoplastic and non-neoplastic entities may arise in the pineal region but originate outside of the pineal gland, evoking a diverse differential diagnosis.

Pineocytoma
Pineocytoma, one of the most common pineal parenchymal tumors, is a slow-growing, well-differentiated WHO grade I neoplasm. Small lesions often are asymptomatic, whereas large ones may cause obstructive hydrocephalus and Parinaud syndrome, defined as upward gaze palsy, pupillary light–near dissociation, and convergence retraction nystagmus.

On imaging, these tumors appear as T2/FLAIR hyperintense, well-defined, round or lobular masses with avid solid or rim enhancement and peripherally displaced calcifications (Fig. 14).[1] Intratumoral hemorrhage and cystic changes may be present. An entirely cystic pineocytoma may be indistinguishable from a non-neoplastic pineal cyst; differentiation may not be clinically significant because small lesions are observed with imaging.

Pineal parenchymal tumor of intermediate differentiation
Pineal parenchymal tumor of intermediate differentiation (PPTID), as the name suggests, is a tumor with intermediate prognosis between pineocytoma, and pineoblastoma PPTID may be designated a WHO grade II or III, although 1 study failed to find correlation with outcome.[24] Compared with pineocytomas, PPTIDs are larger in size, more heterogeneous, and overall more aggressive-appearing (see Fig. 14). Multiple cystic components may be present. Physiologic pineal calcifications may be engulfed or peripherally displaced by the mass. Obstructive hydrocephalus, splaying of the internal cerebral veins, and extension into the tectum, third and lateral ventricles, and thalamus are common.

Papillary tumor of the pineal region
Papillary tumors of the pineal region are rare WHO grade II or grade III neoplasms that do not arise from the pineal gland but from the subcommissural organ of the third ventricle.[1] They are discussed due to their categorization with the primary parenchymal tumors in the 2016 WHO classification. The imaging findings are indistinguishable from those of PPTID.

Meningiomas

Meningiomas are the most common primary intracranial neoplasms. This tumor category includes typical meningiomas, which are benign WHO grade I tumors, and meningioma variants, which include tumors with more aggressive clinical behavior, such as WHO grade II atypical meningiomas and WHO grade III anaplastic meningiomas.[1] Although previously considered a staging feature, brain invasion in the 2016 WHO classification is now considered a grading feature and a histologic criterion, which in itself may establish the diagnosis of WHO grade II atypical meningioma.[4,5]

Typical meningioma
Typical meningiomas account for approximately 95% of all meningiomas.[1] They are benign, WHO grade I tumors most commonly located along the convexity, parasagittal region, or the sphenoid ridge, although they may occur almost anywhere within the CNS (eg, orbits, sinuses, calvarium, ventricles, or pineal region). They are seen most commonly in middle-aged to older adults, with

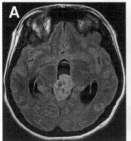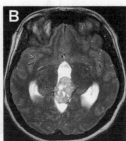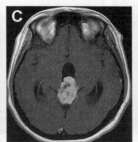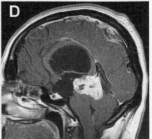

Fig. 14. A PPTID displays heterogeneous signal intensity lesion on axial FLAIR (A) and T2WI (B), heterogeneous enhancement on axial (C) and sagittal (D) postcontrast T1WI, and resultant regional mass effect on the tectal plate with effacement of the cerebral aqueduct and obstructive hydrocephalus.

female predominance. Ionizing radiation is a risk factor. A majority of tumors are asymptomatic, incidental, and indolent. Despite their WHO grade I classification, metastases have been rarely reported.[25]

Typical imaging findings include an extra-axial, dural-based, well-defined, markedly homogeneously enhancing mass (**Fig. 15**A, B). Tumor shape may be round, lobulated, or flat (en plaque). On CT, a vast majority are hyperdense and hyperostosis of the overlying calvarium may be present. Peritumoral edema of the underlying brain parenchyma is present in approximately half of cases irrespective of size or grade.[1] Calcification is seen in one-quarter of cases (see **Fig. 15**C). Intratumoral cysts and hemorrhage are rare. Signal void structures may be present, reflecting tumor vascularity. If present, a dural tail, representing reactive dura, is suggestive of, but not specific for, meningioma.

Atypical meningioma
Atypical meningiomas are WHO grade II tumors diagnosed histologically by the presence of greater than or equal to 4 mitotic figures per high-power field, brain invasion, or on the basis of additive criteria of 3 out of 5 histologic findings.[4] They are associated with higher recurrence rates compared with typical meningiomas.[1]

Unlike typical meningiomas, atypical meningiomas more frequently exhibit ill-defined margins, invasion, and destruction of overlying calvarium or invasion of the underlying parenchyma (**Fig. 16**). The absence of such findings does not exclude atypical meningioma; brain invasion inconspicuous on imaging may be present on histology. Unfortunately, no imaging feature reliably distinguishes typical meningioma from its more aggressive variants, albeit typical meningiomas are statistically far more common. The mushrooming sign, representing tumor extending away from the more central predominant component of the mass, has been associated with higher grade meningiomas.[26]

Anaplastic meningioma
Also known as malignant meningiomas, anaplastic meningiomas are WHO grade III tumors whose diagnosis is based on overt histologic features of malignancy (eg, pleomorphism and high mitotic rates). The prognosis is poor, with low recurrence-free and overall survival rates. Imaging findings overlap with those of atypical meningiomas, including the mushrooming appearance.

Nerve Sheath Tumors

A vast majority of intracranial and skull base nerve sheath tumors are benign, rare (with the exception of vestibular schwannomas), and associated with cranial nerves (CNs). Hybrid nerve sheath tumors (a histologic combination of schwannomas, neurofibromas, and perineuriomas) and melanotic schwannomas have been included as new entities in the 2016 WHO classification.[4] Hybrid nerve sheath tumors are seen more commonly in the body than in the CNS. Two subtypes of malignant peripheral nerve sheath tumors (MPNSTs) now exist: epithelioid MPNSTs and MPNSTs with perineurial differentiation.[4]

Schwannoma
Schwannomas are benign, WHO grade I, slow-growing tumors composed of well-differentiated Schwann cells; they may arise from CN III through CN XII or any peripheral nerve. Approximately 95% of schwannomas arise from CN VIII; CN V is the second most common CN of origin,[1] with involvement of the remaining CNs comprising a small minority of cases. Multinodular or plexiform schwannomas are tumors with multiple

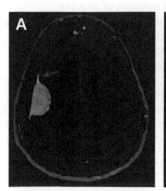 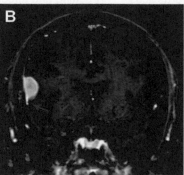 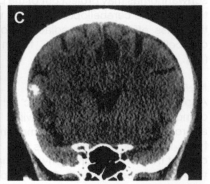

Fig. 15. A right frontoparietal convexity typical meningioma on brain MR imaging shows homogenous enhancement with dural tail (*red arrow*) on axial (*A*) and coronal (*B*) postcontrast T1WI. There are coarse calcifications associated with the tumor as seen on the noncontrast coronal head CT (*C*).

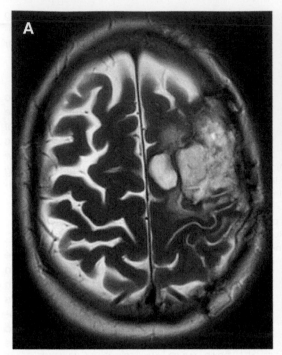
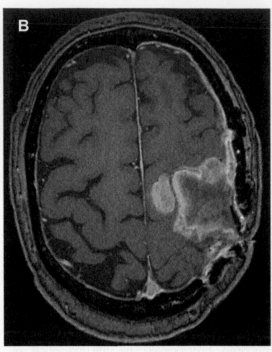

Fig. 16. Atypical meningioma shows irregular margins and invasion of the left frontal and precentral gyrus with associated vasogenic edema (*A*) and irregular enhancement after contrast administration (*B*). There is evidence of prior left frontoparietal craniotomy from prior resection.

consecutive lesions arising along a nerve fascicle along the neck, trunk, and extremities.

Imaging reveals a well-defined extra-axial, T2/FLAIR hyperintense, and avidly homogeneously or heterogeneously enhancing mass near or arising from a CN. In contrast to meningiomas, intratumoral calcification and dural tails are rare, whereas microhemorrhage is characteristic for schwannomas. Approximately 15% of tumors have intratumoral cysts.[1] Small intracanalicular vestibular schwannomas present simply as round or fusiform filling defects within the normal bright CSF on heavily T2WI (**Fig. 17**). Larger vestibular schwannomas may project out of the porus acusticus into the cerebellopontine angle with potential mass effect on the adjacent pons, middle cerebellar peduncle, and fourth ventricle (**Fig. 18**).

Melanotic schwannoma
Approximately 10% of melanotic schwannomas demonstrate malignant behavior. Moreover, approximately 50% of the psammomatous subtype melanotic schwannomas are genetically distinct from conventional schwannomas, in which they are associated with Carney complex and PRKAR1A gene mutation.[27] In light of these findings, melanotic schwannomas are now classified as a distinct entity rather than as a variant.

These tumors most commonly occur in paraspinal and extraneural locations.[1] The presence of melanin accounts for the hyperintense T1 and hypointense T2 signal of these lesions; enhancement is variable.

Neurofibroma
Neurofibromas are WHO grade I neoplasms that can occur anywhere in the dermis or subcutis of the body and rarely along CNs. Multiple neurofibromas and/or plexiform neurofibromas occur in neurofibromatosis type 1 (NF-1). Solitary and sporadic neurofibromas may occur outside of the NF-1 setting and affect patients of all ages.

On imaging, sporadic neurofibromas of the head and neck most frequently present as focal, homogeneously enhancing, well-defined round or ovoid scalp masses that abut and remodel the underlying calvarium (**Fig. 19**A). In contrast, plexiform neurofibromas present as extensive, infiltrating, heterogeneously enhancing soft tissue masses invading and deforming the scalp, parotid gland, or orbit with surround bony remodeling and expansion (see **Fig. 19**B).

Malignant peripheral nerve sheath tumors
MPNSTs are rare malignancies most frequently involving spinal and peripheral nerves, and rarely CNs, arising either de novo or via malignant

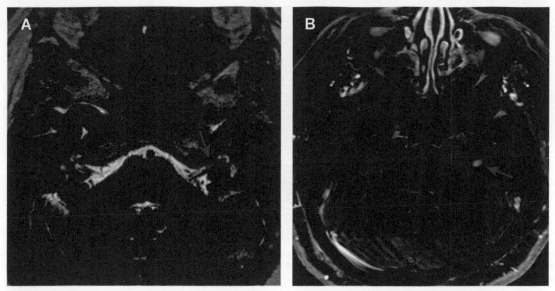

Fig. 17. A small schwannoma is seen as a filling defect on heavily T2 imaging through the internal auditory canals (*red arrow* [*A*]) and homogenously enhances (*red arrow* [*B*]).

degeneration of a neurofibroma. Those arising from a peripheral nerve are strongly associated with NF-1.

Small MPNSTs may be radiologically indistinguishable from schwannomas or sporadic fibromas. Large MPNSTs have similar infiltrating appearances as plexiform neurofibromas but are more likely to demonstrate frank bone invasion and destruction. Sudden rapid enlargement and painfulness of a previous plexiform neurofibroma raises suspicion malignant degeneration. The optimal way to distinguish between MPNSTs from the benign counterpart is with 2-deoxy-2-(18F)fluoro-D-glucose PET where a standardized uptake value of greater than 3 indicates MPNST.[28]

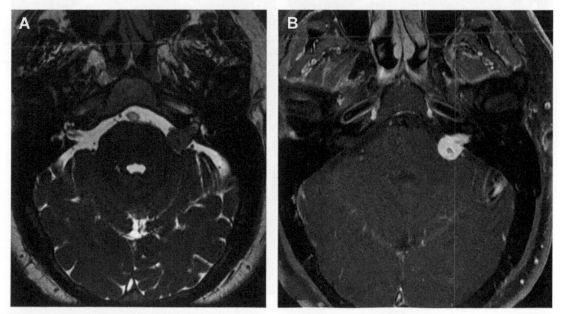

Fig. 18. A large schwannoma shows slight T2 hyperintensity on heavily T2-weighted sequence through the internal auditory canal (*A*) and near-complete homogenous enhancement (*B*). There is a focus of hypoenhancement in the lesion representing cystic degenerative change.

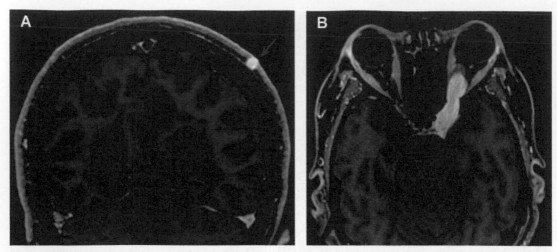

Fig. 19. A patient with a left parietal small scalp neurofibroma is seen on the coronal postcontrast image (*red arrow* [*A*]). A postcontrast axial T1 in a different patient shows a homogenously enhancing neurofibroma of left CN III (*B*).

Lymphoma and Mesenchymal Tumors

Expansion of entities in the classification of systemic lymphomas over the past decade has been followed by similar updates in 2016 CNS WHO classification.[4] Greater than 95% of CNS lymphomas, however, remain diffuse large B-cell lymphomas, which are the specific type discussed in this article.[1] A brief discussion of a particular mesenchymal tumor, solitary fibrous tumors (SFTs), is also provided, given changes in the 2016 WHO classification.

Diffuse large B-cell lymphoma
On imaging, up to three-fourths of diffuse large B-cell lymphomas contact the CSF via the ependymal or pial surface.[1] Periventricular white matter and deep gray nuclei are the most common locations; involvement of the subependyma and corpus callosum is not infrequent. Lesions

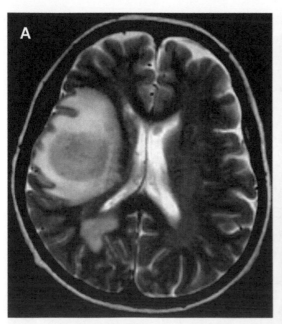
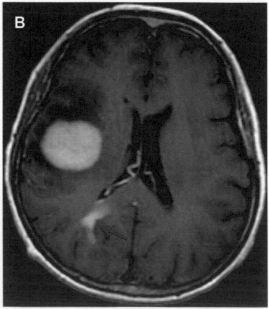

Fig. 20. Diffuse large B-cell lymphoma in this immunocompetent patient exhibits heterogeneous right corona radiata lesion with extensive vasogenic edema (*A*) and homogenous enhancement (*B*). There is a smaller heterogeneous T2 lesion (*A*) in the right splenium of the corpus callosum that homogenously enhances (*red arrow* [*B*]) and represents a satellite tumor.

characteristically homogenously enhance, restrict on DWI, and are hyperdense on CT (**Fig. 20**), correlating to the densely packed cells angiocentric pattern of tumor cells within and around blood vessels. By comparison, multifocality, necrosis, ring or heterogeneous enhancement, and intratumoral hemorrhage may be seen in immunocompromised patients, including those with human immunodeficiency virus, making such tumors indistinguishable from glioblastoma on imaging.

Solitary fibrous tumor/hemangiopericytoma

It is now apparent that SFTs and hemangiopericytomas are very similar, if not the same entity.[29,30] Neuropathologists now join the rest of soft tissue pathologists in using the term, *SFT*, but retain the term, *hemangiopericytoma*, to create the combined moniker, *SFT/hemangiopericytoma*, for continuity. SFTs represent a continuum of mesenchymal tumors with varying cellularity notorious for their aggressive behavior, recurrence, and metastases, which may be designated WHO grade I, II, or III.

Low-grade SFTs are well-defined, extra-axial, dural-based, heterogeneously intense, avidly enhancing masses that mimic typical meningiomas and most commonly occur at the posterior falx or tentorium. High-grade SFTs mimic aggressive meningiomas; however, dural tails, hyperostosis, and intratumoral calcification typically are absent.

SUMMARY

The unprecedented use of molecular parameters and creation of genetically defined parameters to establish brain tumor diagnoses in the 2016 WHO classification is a major paradigm shift. Major paradigm restructuring resulted in classifying diffuse gliomas, such as astrocytomas, oligodendrogliomas, and glioblastomas, as genetically defined entities. Molecular markers not only are of diagnostic significance but also are of prognostic value. These more objectively defined entities allow for more accurate diagnoses, therapies, stratification, and recruitment within clinical trials, and categorization in epidemiologic studies. Imaging remains a mainstay modality in the diagnosis and management of these entities, and familiarity with the new classification scheme, therefore, is crucial for neuroradiologists to communicate meaningfully with radiation oncologists, neuropathologists, neuro-oncologists, and neurosurgeons.

REFERENCES

1. Osborn AG, Hedlund GL, Salzman KL. Osborn's brain. 2nd edition. Salt Lake City (UT): Elsevier; 2018.

2. Ostrom QT, Gittleman H, Truitt G, et al. CBTRUS statistical report: primary brain and other central nervous system tumors diagnosed in the United States in 2011-2015. Neuro Oncol 2018;20(suppl_4):iv1–86.

3. Komori T. The 2016 WHO classification of tumours of the central nervous system: the major points of revision. Neurol Med Chir (Tokyo) 2017;57(7):301–11.

4. Louis DN, Perry A, Reifenberger G, et al. The 2016 World Health Organization classification of tumors of the central nervous system: a summary. Acta Neuropathol 2016;131(6):803–20.

5. Banan R, Hartmann C. The new WHO 2016 classification of brain tumors-what neurosurgeons need to know. Acta Neurochir (Wien) 2017;159(3):403–18.

6. Louis DN, Wesseling P, Paulus W, et al. cIMPACT-NOW update 1: not otherwise specified (NOS) and not elsewhere classified (NEC). Acta Neuropathol 2018;135(3):481–4.

7. Bielle F, Di Stefano AL, Meyronet D, et al. Diffuse gliomas with FGFR3-TACC3 fusion have characteristic histopathological and molecular features. Brain Pathol 2018;28(5):674–83.

8. Johnson DR, Guerin JB, Giannini C, et al. 2016 updates to the WHO brain tumor classification system: what the radiologist needs to know. Radiographics 2017;37(7):2164–80.

9. van den Bent MJ, Brandes AA, Taphoorn MJ, et al. Adjuvant procarbazine, lomustine, and vincristine chemotherapy in newly diagnosed anaplastic oligodendroglioma: long-term follow-up of EORTC brain tumor group study 26951. J Clin Oncol 2013;31(3):344–50.

10. Cairncross JG, Wang M, Jenkins RB, et al. Benefit from procarbazine, lomustine, and vincristine in oligodendroglial tumors is associated with mutation of IDH. J Clin Oncol 2014;32(8):783–90.

11. Buckner JC, Shaw EG, Pugh SL, et al. Radiation plus procarbazine, CCNU, and vincristine in low-grade glioma. N Engl J Med 2016;374(14):1344–55.

12. Weller M, Weber RG, Willscher E, et al. Molecular classification of diffuse cerebral WHO grade II/III gliomas using genome- and transcriptome-wide profiling improves stratification of prognostically distinct patient groups. Acta Neuropathol 2015;129(5):679–93.

13. Suzuki H, Aoki K, Chiba K, et al. Mutational landscape and clonal architecture in grade II and III gliomas. Nat Genet 2015;47(5):458–68.

14. Olar A, Wani KM, Alfaro-Munoz KD, et al. IDH mutation status and role of WHO grade and mitotic index in overall survival in grade II-III diffuse gliomas. Acta Neuropathol 2015;129(4):585–96.

15. Saito T, Muragaki Y, Maruyama T, et al. Calcification on CT is a simple and valuable preoperative indicator of 1p/19q loss of heterozygosity in supratentorial

brain tumors that are suspected grade II and III gliomas. Brain Tumor Pathol 2016;33(3):175–82.

16. Kleinschmidt-DeMasters BK, Mulcahy Levy JM. H3 K27M-mutant gliomas in adults vs. children share similar histological features and adverse prognosis. Clin Neuropathol 2018;37 (2018)(2):53–63.

17. Ebrahimi A, Skardelly M, Schuhmann MU, et al. High frequency of H3 K27M mutations in adult midline gliomas. J Cancer Res Clin Oncol 2019;145(4):839–50.

18. Louis DN, Giannini C, Capper D, et al. cIMPACT-NOW update 2: diagnostic clarifications for diffuse midline glioma, H3 K27M-mutant and diffuse astrocytoma/anaplastic astrocytoma, IDH-mutant. Acta Neuropathol 2018;135(4):639–42.

19. Tihan T, Zhou T, Holmes E, et al. The prognostic value of histological grading of posterior fossa ependymomas in children: a Children's Oncology Group study and a review of prognostic factors. Mod Pathol 2008;21(2):165–77.

20. Pajtler KW, Witt H, Sill M, et al. Molecular classification of ependymal tumors across all CNS compartments, histopathological grades, and age groups. Cancer Cell 2015;27(5):728–43.

21. Mack SC, Witt H, Piro RM, et al. Epigenomic alterations define lethal CIMP-positive ependymomas of infancy. Nature 2014;506(7489):445–50.

22. Parker M, Mohankumar KM, Punchihewa C, et al. C11orf95-RELA fusions drive oncogenic NF-kappaB signalling in ependymoma. Nature 2014;506(7489):451–5.

23. Yang C, Fang J, Li G, et al. Histopathological, molecular, clinical and radiological characterization of rosette-forming glioneuronal tumor in the central nervous system. Oncotarget 2017;8(65):109175–90.

24. Yu T, Sun X, Wang J, et al. Twenty-seven cases of pineal parenchymal tumours of intermediate differentiation: mitotic count, Ki-67 labelling index and extent of resection predict prognosis. J Neurol Neurosurg Psychiatry 2016;87(4):386–95.

25. Simonetti G, Terreni MR, DiMeco F, et al. Letter to the editor: lung metastasis in WHO grade I meningioma. Neurol Sci 2018;39(10):1781–3.

26. Shapir J, Coblentz C, Malanson D, et al. New CT finding in aggressive meningioma. AJNR Am J Neuroradiol 1985;6(1):101–2.

27. Carney JA. Psammomatous melanotic schwannoma. A distinctive, heritable tumor with special associations, including cardiac myxoma and the Cushing syndrome. Am J Surg Pathol 1990;14(3):206–22.

28. Vezina G. Neuroimaging of phakomatoses: overview and advances. Pediatr Radiol 2015;45(Suppl 3):S433–42.

29. Robinson DR, Wu YM, Kalyana-Sundaram S, et al. Identification of recurrent NAB2-STAT6 gene fusions in solitary fibrous tumor by integrative sequencing. Nat Genet 2013;45(2):180–5.

30. Chmielecki J, Crago AM, Rosenberg M, et al. Whole-exome sequencing identifies a recurrent NAB2-STAT6 fusion in solitary fibrous tumors. Nat Genet 2013;45(2):131–2.

Moving?

Make sure your subscription moves with you!

To notify us of your new address, find your **Clinics Account Number** (located on your mailing label above your name), and contact customer service at:

Email: journalscustomerservice-usa@elsevier.com

800-654-2452 (subscribers in the U.S. & Canada)
314-447-8871 (subscribers outside of the U.S. & Canada)

Fax number: 314-447-8029

Elsevier Health Sciences Division
Subscription Customer Service
3251 Riverport Lane
Maryland Heights, MO 63043

Printed and bound by CPI Group (UK) Ltd, Croydon, CR0 4YY

03/10/2024

01040372-0013